Medical Genetics

Its Application to Speech, Hearing, and Craniofacial Disorders

Genetic Syndromes and Communication Disorders Series

Robert J. Shprintzen, Ph.D.
Series Editor

Waardenburg Syndrome by Alice Kahn, Ph.D.
Educating Children with Velo-Cardio-Facial Syndrome
by Donna Cutler-Landsman, M.S., Editor

Medical Genetics

Its Application to Speech, Hearing, and Craniofacial Disorders

A Volume in the
Genetics and Communication Disorders Series

Nathaniel H. Robin, M.D.

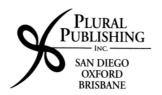

PLURAL
PUBLISHING
— INC. —
SAN DIEGO
OXFORD
BRISBANE

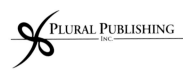

PLURAL PUBLISHING
INC.

5521 Ruffin Road
San Diego, CA 92123

e-mail: info@pluralpublishing.com
Web site: http://www.pluralpublishing.com

49 Bath Street
Abingdon, Oxfordshire OX14 1EA
United Kingdom

Typeset in 11/13 [Garamond] by Flanagan's Publishing Services, Inc.
Printed in Hong Kong by Paramount Printing.

For permission to use material from this text, contact us by
Telephone: (866) 758-7251
Fax: (888) 758-7255
e-mail: permissions@pluralpublishing.com

*Every attempt has been made to contact the copyright holders for material origi-
nally printed in another source. If any have been inadvertently overlooked, the
publishers will gladly make the necessary arrangements at the first opportunity.*

Library of Congress Cataloging-in-Publication Data:
Robin, Nathaniel.
    Medical genetics / by Nathaniel Robin.
        p. ; cm. — (Genetic syndromes and communication disorders series)
    Includes bibliographical references.
    ISBN-13: 978-1-59756-258-4 (pbk.)
    ISBN-10: 1-59756-258-0 (pbk.)
    1. Medical genetics. I. Title. II. Series.
    [DNLM: 1. Genetics, Medical. 2. Genetic Diseases, Inborn. 3. Genetic
Screening. QZ 50 R655m 2007]
    RB155.R656 2007
    616'.042–dc22
                                                            2007036511

Contents

Foreword

*T*his volume is meant to serve as an introduction to the field of genomics for professionals who see children with congenital anomalies, yet who may have little familiarity with the meaning of those anomalies and the role they play in overall development over time. Although genomics now encompasses many thousands of practitioners around the world, some disciplines have been slow to recognize the importance of the genetic code and have not updated their curricula to reflect its overall importance in the health care field. The communication sciences, in particular, have been left behind by other behavioral fields in bringing its practitioners to the state-of-the-art. This volume will be an important first step in introducing the reader to the fascinating field of human genomics.

The science of genomics, how variations in the genetic code that exists in each and every one of us, has advanced at such a rapid pace over the past two decades that "old-timers" like myself who remember the science we used to call syndromology in the 1970s find little resemblance to current practices in medical genetics. Microdeletion syndromes, upstream and downstream gene-to-gene interactions, imprinting, anticipation, and other topics commonly discussed today were not even in our lexicon at the time. It is not without some struggle that those of us who cut our teeth on identifying abnormal patterns of anomalies back then try to keep pace with this next generation of scientists and clinicians who are conversant with both laboratory and clinical aspects of genetic disorders. If we are fortunate, we are able to plot the advancement of science through the eyes of those we have had a hand in training. I had the good fortune to play a small role in education of Nathaniel Robin (whom I will call Nat from here forward) in the early 1990s while he was a pediatric resident at Montefiore Medical Center and the Albert Einstein College of Medicine in the Bronx. Nat dove into a rotation in the craniofacial program that I directed at the time with such enthusiasm and aplomb that it became obvious to me that he would become a prominent and driving force in the field. He did not disappoint. He is now training the next generation of genetic specialists knowing so much more than I could even dream about a generation ago. Nat knows his way around a DNA molecule as well as he examines the human body. He has reached out to professionals from many fields, including the communication sciences, and I have learned that he knows how to speak our language. When Plural Publishing took the bold action of becoming a driving force, if not the primary force in bringing this science to its readership, it became obvious that an introductory volume was sorely needed. As Series Editor, I had to select an author who was an expert without being pedantic. Nat filled this bill perfectly. The reader can look forward to getting a superb education in human genetics within a volume that is easy to read while being genuinely authoritative.

Robert J. Shprintzen, Ph.D.
Professor of Otolaryngology
Professor of Pediatrics
Director, Communication Disorder Unit
Director, Velo-Cardio-Facial Syndrome
   International Center
Director, Center for Genetic
   Communicative Disorders
Upstate Medical University
Syracuse, New York
Series Editor

Preface

We are in the age of genetics in medicine. Thanks to the Human Genome Project, genetic discoveries are occurring at a rapid rate. Medical journals are dominated by papers that announce the discovery of the latest disease-related genes, and new genetic tests are entering clinical practice. This enthusiasm is not limited to the scientific arena, as genetics is a frequent topic in the popular press and mass media. Magazine stories, television shows and movies have all feature genetic topics prominently.

While this exposure has in many ways been exciting, it has in general portrayed genetics and genetic technology as having powers that is neither accurate nor realistic. This has had the unintended result of having the public either fearing genetics, or expecting it to solve all medical ills. Furthermore, it has lead to confusion between the science of genetics and the medical specialty of genetics, which is the topic of this book.

The science of genetics is the study of heredity. At its most basic level, geneticists study the structure and function of genes, how they work, or fail to work. Medical genetics is, on the other hand, a medical discipline whose focus is the evaluation and management of patients with a genetically determined disorder, and their families. Unlike the science of genetics, medical genetics has a low profile. Few people know it even exists. This includes not only the lay public but other physicians and other healthcare providers. There are many reasons for this – there are relatively few medical geneticists, and we are typically found at large medical centers. And we care for patients with rare, often esoteric diseases. However, while I am not surprised that so few know what I do, I have always been surprised the colleagues who I interact with regarding these patients really do not know what a geneticist does.

To address this problem I have made it a personal mission to educate my colleagues about my field. I do this for two reasons. The first is based on the belief that as people learn about my field they will recognize the potential benefits a genetics evaluation has to offer. They will then be quicker to refer patients. The second reason is less practical. I find medical genetics an extremely interesting field, and I love to talk about it. Medical geneticists are also very old fashioned in much of what we do. With apologies to the CSI shows, we are the last medical detectives, searching for tiny clues to make a diagnosis.

At the same time, we utilize the most modern technologies of genetic testing. We are a field at the intersection of a very complex and rapidly advancing basic science and clinical care. Furthermore, we often encounter situations that call into play ethical and legal issues. It is, to be frank, a lot of fun.

Medical geneticists are, at our core, educators. We explain difficult genetic concepts to our patients, our students, and our peers. I give well over 100 lectures and talks per year to every type of audience, not only medically trained but other healthcare professionals as well as the lay public. So when I was asked by my friend and mentor, Dr. Robert Shprintzen, to write a book on medical genetics I was eager to accept. There are many excellent texts on medical genetics, but few that focus on clinical application of the field. Furthermore, as this book would be part of a series intended for speech-language pathologists and audiologists, I recognized that it would fill an important niche. As you will see, the text is very much oriented to these professionals.

The book's organization echoes the education theme, as it follow a series of lectures that I have given to various healthcare professionals over the years. The chapters are, of course, more detailed, if somewhat less entertaining. Topics were conceived to address questions that I frequently encounter. For example, I know that many people are confused as to what training a medical geneticist receives, and how that is different from a genetic counselor, or someone running a lab. This is covered in Chapter 2. Basic principles and tools of medical genetics are the topics of Chapters 3 through 6. How do you make a genetic diagnosis? Why do we care so much about minor things, like odd creases on the palm? What is cytogenetic testing? Later chapters cover the ethical principles on which the discipline of medical genetics is based, as well as the genetic counseling process. The last three chapters can be considered as a single theme, with different units. Each provides an overview on the genetics evaluation to a specific type of patient that is commonly encountered by an audiologist or speech and language pathologist—hearing impairment (Chapter 9), orofacial clefting (Chapter 10), and craniofacial anomalies, including craniosynostosis (Chapter 11). These are not, of course, intended to be all inclusive or highly detailed, but rather review common disorders as well as provide a framework in which to view each patient.

At the end of each chapter is a list of additional reading. This is to guide the reader to more detailed source, as this is not meant to be viewed as an authorative reference text. Rather, it was written in a conversational tone that was meant to mimic my lectures on these topics, and hopefully to allow the material to be more easily understood. At the end, I hope you will share, or at least understand, my enthusiasm for this fascinating field.

Acknowledgments

As with any major effort, this book could not have been done without the help and assistance of many other people. First and foremost, I would like to thank my assistant Sandra Pilkinton. Her tireless assistance in editing, organizing, and everything else made this book possible (and kept me sane).

Many people took time to critically read sections of the book, and provided important comments, edits, and advice. Several who provided especially valuable feedback are Dr. Richard JH Smith, the Director of the Molecular Otolaryngology Research Laboratories at the University of Iowa; Drs. Lane Rutledge, Fady Mikail, and Andrew Carroll, all colleagues of mine in the University of Alabama at Birmingham's Department of Genetics; Judy Mann and Elizabeth Baker, both speech and language pathologists for the University of Alabama at Birmingham's Cleft and Craniofacial Clinics; Heather Baty, the head of audiology at The Children's Hospital of Alabama; and Dr. John Grant, the Plastic Surgeon and Director of that clinic. Dr. Grant, along with Dr. Raoul Hennekam, a noted medical geneticist at Great Ormond Street in London, and Judy Franklin, a genetics nurse at UAB, provided many of the clinical images in the book.

My deepest gratitude to Dr. Robert Shprintzen, the director of the Center for the Diagnosis, Treatment, and Study of Velo-Cardio-Facial Syndrome Center for Genetic Communicative Disorders Communication Disorder Unit at Upstate Medical University in Syracuse, New York. Since my days as a pediatric resident, Dr. Shprintzen has been a mentor to me as well as a friend. I was honored that he considered me to write this contribution to his series. He was instrumental in the completion of this book in many ways. He provided clinical images and editorial suggestions, and he was willing to write the foreword.

Lastly, I must thank my family—my wife Laurie, my sons Joseph (it is his head in Figure 1–3A), Timmy, and Alex—for their support in this and all my efforts.

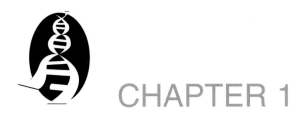

CHAPTER 1

Introduction

*H*ereditary factors play an important role in causing human diseases. Although this has been recognized for centuries, genetics as a scientific field has been in existence for only about 100 years. As a medical specialty, genetics is far younger, just over 50 years old. In that time, medical geneticists have made great strides in recognizing and categorizing birth defects and genetic syndromes. More recently, the remarkable explosion of genetic research has expanded our knowledge about the genetic basis of many of these disorders as well as many common diseases, such as hearing impairment and clefting. Furthermore, diseases such as autism and language impairment that were once thought to be too complex to ever be understood at the basic genetic level are now being investigated using incredibly sophisticated new technologies, such as expression arrays that can look at the activity of hundreds of genes simultaneously. Although years away, it is expected that this research will one day provide clinically useful genetic information for these patients in the form of new genetic tests and treatments that are aimed at the basic underlying cause.

It is evident that genetics is at the forefront of medicine. However, for many health care providers and members of the lay public, genetics is viewed as a research field whose sole purpose is to find and study new disease-related genes. Although such research is certainly one important facet of genetics, genetics is a far broader field that includes a clinical branch. With many different subspecialties and a wide range of professionals serving a very diverse patient population, medical (or clinical) genetics is a small but very active medical specialty.

Historically, medical genetics has focused on pediatric patients, those with inherited and congenital anomalies. As such, genetics is well known to most professionals who care for pediatric-age patients. The purpose of these evaluations was to make a diagnosis of a genetic syndrome (see Benefits of

Making a Diagnosis). Some syndromes are well known, such as Down syndrome, but most are rare disorders with strange names. Often, tests are ordered that are unusual and complex with results that are an incomprehensible amalgam of letters and numbers. To most health care professionals, the geneticist's evaluation of a patient, the tests that are ordered, and the method by which a diagnosis is made, are a "black box" (Figure 1–1): a patient goes in with a complex array of problems and emerges with a single unifying diagnosis but the process is not understood.

This is, of course, an oversimplification, and it is inaccurate. Even in the hands of the best clinical geneticist, a diagnosis cannot be made for most patients. This does not diminish the fact that every effort should be made to make a diagnosis, because it is very significant if one is reached. However, the process by which a genetics evaluation is carried out is indeed a mystery to most health care providers. This can have several untoward effects. For one, not knowing what a geneticist offers may mean that appropriate referrals are not made. Most health care providers know that clinical geneticists evaluate children with birth defects, developmental disability, or an abnormal facial appearance. However, research is increasing our understanding of the contribution of genetic factors to a wide variety of diseases, and therefore expanding the types of patients that would benefit from a genetics evaluation. Hearing impairment is one such example. It has long been recognized that a substantial proportion of hearing impairment is genetic. However, the benefit of a genetics evaluation for a child with hearing impairment was minimal. Through taking detailed medical and family histories and performing a specialized physical examination, a geneticist would determine if the hearing impairment was one component manifestation of a genetic syndrome, or if it was isolated. Counseling could then be provided for cases of syndromic hearing impairment. However, unless there was a family history that suggested a specific inheritance pattern; there was little to offer for isolated hearing

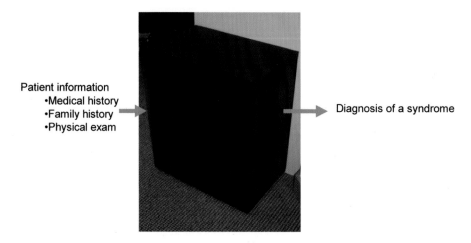

Patient information
•Medical history
•Family history
•Physical exam

Diagnosis of a syndrome

FIGURE 1–1. The medical genetics evaluation.

impairment beyond empiric recurrence risk estimates. Today, thanks to the significant progress in genetic research made in the past decade, genetic testing is an integral part of the evaluation of hearing impairment. This is one example, but there are many others where genetic research has led to discoveries that have expanded the practice of clinical genetics. Coronary artery disease, diabetes, and hypertension are examples of common diseases with a strong genetic influence, and for each there are ongoing active research efforts. It is expected that genetic testing will be available in the near future, which will further expand the list of conditions that are seen by a geneticist. However, regardless of the type of disease, the clinical geneticist's evaluation remains essentially unchanged.

The Benefits of Making the Diagnosis of a Genetic Syndrome

We are in the age of genetics, as genetic research is transforming our understanding of many diseases. Such advances are occurring in cancer, cardiac disease, and hearing loss, transforming our understanding of the basic causes of these diseases. Referred to as "Genomic Medicine," this promises new and improved diagnostic tests and an enhanced understanding of disease process that will lead to better treatments and quality of life for children affected with these diseases. Although many view Genomic Medicine as "new," it is in fact no different than what medical geneticists have always done. Genomic Medicine represents only an expansion of what we medical geneticists have always provided in activities like syndrome identification. Many have viewed this activity as unnecessary— placing a unifying name to a child's medical problems had limited value. This was exemplified to me when, as a young attending I evaluated a hospitalized young child because one of his doctors suspected that the child had a genetic syndrome. He had several congenital anomalies, and what they perceived was a distinctive facial appearance—the child looked "different." He had been admitted for evaluation of poor weight gain, but as I learned later he was also developmentally delayed, and his mother had had a cleft palate repaired as a young child. She also had learning disabilities, and had battled depression most of her life. The diagnosis was quickly evident—the child, and the mother, had deletion 22q11 (Del22q11) syndrome. Also known as Shprintzen syndrome or velocardiofacial syndrome (VCFS), which is one of the most common genetic syndromes seen in cleft centers. It is associated with a wide variety of medical, developmental, and behavioral problems.

When I told the team about my diagnosis, one of the medical students challenged me, asking me what good will come of making that diagnosis? I had heard comments like that before many times in reference to medical genetics. "All you do is label some kid with one of those strange syndrome names. How does that really help the patient?" This question can be summed up by saying that, to some, a genetic diagnosis is "nice to know," but not something that anyone "needs to know" to help the patient. This notion, however, is in error.

This child had undergone a number of tests as an outpatient at considerable expense and inconvenience to the family. I met with the house staff team, discussed my diagnosis, and told how this diagnosis not only explained the facial appearance but also the poor weight gain and feeding problems. Children with Del22q11 syndrome commonly have palatal anomalies, ranging from overt or submucous cleft palate to a hypotonic and poorly functioning palate. I went on to describe the natural history of the disease, associated problems, and genetics. Several days later, once the genetic testing had confirmed my clinical diagnosis, I met with the parents to discuss the diagnosis of Del22q11 syndrome. Although understandably upset at the prospect of having a child with medical problems and limited development, the mother also expressed relief. She explained that she had tried everything to get the child to eat, but nothing worked. She felt incredibly guilty and inadequate, and had become distraught at the prospect of being labeled an unfit mother and losing her child. So, although the diagnosis was certainly not "good news," it at least showed that the child's problems were not due to her inadequacies. Furthermore, having the diagnosis meant no more unnecessary tests, and that more accurate anticipatory guidance was possible.

As illustrated by this case, making a genetic diagnosis is far more than an academic exercise. It has many clear benefits for the patient, their family, and the medical team caring for the child. These include:

- **Prognosis.** A correct diagnosis enables accurate prognostic information to be provided to the family. For example, what is the prognosis for a child with a cleft palate? If isolated, it is excellent. A cleft palate is typically repaired at about 9 months of age, and, although such children are at risk for speech problems and maxillofacial growth disturbances, the vast majority will have a favorable outcome. However, the prognosis is likely to be much different if the cleft palate is part of a genetic syndrome. About 25% of cleft palate is seen as one component manifestation of a genetic syndrome, including disorders such as Trisomy 13 or Del 22q11 syndrome. The vast majority of infants with Trisomy 13 die in infancy, and those who survive are severely impaired, with little developmental progress, and they often have many other major medical problems, such as congenital heart defects and seizures. Del22q11 syndrome is associated with other medical problems, such as hypocalcemia, immune dysfunction, and conotruncal heart defects in infancy, and speech problems and learning disabilities later in childhood. Adults have a very elevated (33%) risk for developing a psychiatric disease, such as depression and schizophrenia.

■ **Management.** It is therefore obvious how the prognosis for a given problem can vary considerably based on the correct genetic diagnosis, and issues with management are similarly very different depending on the nature of the genetic diagnosis. A child with a cleft palate often will have feeding problems, requiring a feeding specialist and a special nipple. They usually will have myringotomy tubes placed prophylactically to ensure normal hearing, as recurrent otitis media is a common complication of cleft palate. After palatoplasty (repair of the cleft palate), which usually occurs at about 9 months of age, regular speech pathology evaluations, hearing tests, and dental evaluations are done to ensure normal speech and orofacial growth. However, if the cleft palate is part of Trisomy 13, or Del22q11, the management plans will be quite different. Most infants with Trisomy 13 receive only supportive care, as the likelihood of early death is so very high. For VCFS, surgical plans are different than for isolated cleft palate, as are the rehabilitation plans. These children require more aggressive speech therapy, as there is a greater likelihood of residual speech problems than for nonsyndromic cleft palate. Furthermore, the risk of associated medical problems necessitates additional screenings.

■ **Recurrence risk.** At some point, parents will ask what their chances are of having another child with cleft palate. Such information cannot be provided unless an accurate diagnosis has been made. For an isolated cleft palate born to healthy parents with no family history of cleft palate or related anomalies, the likelihood that a subsequent child will have a cleft palate is about 1%. However, that figure may be drastically different if the cleft palate is syndromic. For Del22q11 syndrome, for example, about 12% of cases are familial. In such cases, the likelihood of a future child having Del22q11 syndrome is 50%, including more severe manifestations, such as life-threatening congenital heart defect or immune dysfunction. If neither parent is affected, which can be determined through genetic testing, the likelihood for an affected offspring is much lower, under 1%.

■ **Why?** Parents will also wonder what caused their child to be born with a cleft. Many will incorrectly attribute the cleft palate to prenatal exposures that have no contributing role, such as dental x-rays or a glass of wine, resulting in parental guilt. By discussing the origin of the birth defect at a scientific level, such feelings can be at least mitigated to some degree. It is important to recognize that this is true not only for genetic syndromes, but for nonsyndromic instances as well. However, the discussions obviously are very different if the birth defect is part of a genetic syndrome.

■ **Access to support groups.** This is an underappreciated aspect of making a genetic diagnosis, but one that nonetheless is of significant importance to parents. As pediatricians we can provide the most current medical care for our patients. However, we cannot know what it is like to be a parent of a child with a genetic syndrome. Although many issues are common to a group of conditions, such as dwarfs or those with mental retardation, many more are specific to a particular disorder. Furthermore, there are opportunities for children with a particular disorder, such as the camps for children with Prader-Willi syndrome. However, to take advantage of these opportunities, one must have been correctly diagnosed with Prader-Willi Syndrome.

■ **Treatments.** Although there are no true cures, a few genetic diseases have therapies that correct the underlying defect. For example, Fabry disease is a disorder in which the enzyme ceramide trihexosidase is defective. Today, this deficiency can be corrected with replacement enzyme in the form of the medication Fabrazyme. Other genetic syndromes have treatments that improve health, such as Osteogenesis Imperfecta (brittle bone disease), which is now treated with bisphosphonates. This family of medications improves bone strength, thereby lessening pain and the rate of fracture.

However, the use of these medications is not possible if an accurate and correct diagnosis is not made. Furthermore, it is not limited to medications. In Fragile X syndrome and Del22q11, for example, studies have shown that certain medications and therapies have greater efficacy in treating the associated problems.

■ **Reduction of cost.** Last, but by no means the least important, is the cost of medical care. Not only does making a correct genetic diagnosis improve medical management by permitting more targeted testing and evaluations, it also obviates the need for unnecessary diagnostic tests. In this manner, a correct genetic diagnosis saves not only money but also inconvenience to patients and their families. For example, one study found that the cost of the evaluation of children with Williams syndrome, a particular syndrome that features developmental delay and other medial complications, was significantly lower once a geneticist was consulted, owing to fewer unnecessary diagnostic tests.

A BRIEF HISTORY OF GENETICS IN MEDICINE

Medical genetics is a relatively new discipline. It was formally recognized in 1993, making it the most recent addition to the list of recognized specialties. However, its origins can be traced back to the mid-19th century to the experiments of an Austrian monk, Gregor Mendel, that lead to the laws of segregation of traits among progeny. These are the principles on which Mendelian inheritance (discussed in Chapter 3) are based.

Mendel's publications were largely ignored at the time, but then rediscovered in the early 20th century. At this time, many scientists made significant discoveries about genetics, such as the identification of chromosomes, and the postulate that chromosomes were the material that passed down the traits in the manner Mendel described. Most of this early work was in plant and animal genetics. Human genetic research was mainly population studies, using biostatistical models. However, several disorders were recognized to follow Mendelian inheritance, such as brachydactyly type A (a form of short fingers; Figure 1-2), and albinism.

Unfortunately, in the early 20th century the new science of genetics was used to support the eugenics movement. This was intended to improve the human race by eradicating "bad genes." To achieve that goal, societies around

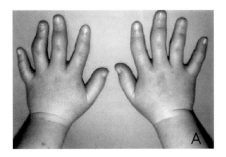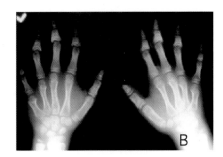

FIGURE 1–2. Brachydactyly type A. This was one of the first physical anomalies recognized to have a Mendelian inheritance (autosomal dominant) pattern. **A.** The dorsal view of this 10-year-old child's hands demonstrates generally short digits, most apparent in the middle phalanges, and variable radial and ulnar clinodactyly. **B.** Radiographs demonstrate the shortness most apparent in all of the middle phalanges as well as the proximal and distal phalanges, and the fourth and fifth metacarpals. (Reprinted with permission from the *British Medical Journal* from "Clinical and Radiologic Assessment of a Family with Mild Brachydactyly Type AI: The Usefulness of Metacarpophalangeal Profiles," by C. M. Armour, D. E., Bulman, & A. G. Hunter, 2000. *Journal of Medical Genetics, 37,* 292–296.)

the world, including the United States, intended to limit the reproduction of those with undesirable traits, like mental or physical defects, through programs such as forced sterilization. Unfortunately it was this movement that influenced those who perpetrated the atrocities carried out by the Nazis in World War II.

With the specter of eugenics lingering, the community of genetic scientists formed the American Society of Human Genetics in 1948. Stringent ethical principles were written into the bylaws (http://www.ashg.org), but the field of genetics was at that time a research field with few physicians as members. However, a clinical interest soon developed, focused primarily on genetic diseases of childhood. This included both direct patient care as well as clinical laboratory activities.

Initially, patient care focused on children with birth defects. Soon after, prenatal genetic counseling grew as a second major area of clinical genetics. This was made possible by the ability to perform accurate and rapid tests that could assess the status of a developing fetus. These included maternal serum screening and chromosome analysis on cells obtained through another new technique, amniocentesis.

The scope of genetics in medicine remained largely unchanged for many years, as clinical genetics was synonymous with pediatric syndrome identification and prenatal genetic testing and counseling. This has begun now to change, with the explosion of genetic information in the past decade, and with it a vast array of new genetic tests. Today, clinical genetics is expanding to be involved in the care of all types of patients.

DYSMORPHOLOGY AND GENOMIC MEDICINE

Although one of the older aspects of clinical genetics, syndrome identification, is still a relatively new field. Individuals had for many years tried to understand birth defects, but it was through development of a unified approach, called dysmorphology, in which the greatest strides were made. Dysmorphology refers to the study of abnormal form. The clinical application of the dysmorphologic examination is to identify an underlying syndrome to explain the patient's abnormalities. Dysmorphology is a term that was coined by David W. Smith, one of the earliest physicians to begin to scientifically categorize and classify patients with physical and cognitive abnormalities. This systematic approach related the observed anomaly back to an underlying abnormality in embryogenesis. His landmark book, *Smith's Recognizable Patterns of Human Malformations,* (commonly referred to as "*Smith's*") remains the primary resource for syndrome identification for geneticists, pediatricians, and any other health care providers for children. *Smith's* also provides an excellent review of the approach to the evaluation of a patient with a developmental abnormality, including the special features of the physical exam.

As we discuss in more detail in Chapter 4, the genetic physical exam is characterized by careful observation of physical landmarks, especially subtle findings that other physicians would ignore. Hair pattern, spacing between the eyes, creases on the palm (Figures 1–3A, 1–3B, and 1–3C) are examples of minor findings that have no impact on the patient's medical status, but may lead to the identification of a genetic syndrome.

Syndrome identification is the traditional role for clinical geneticists in the care of a patient with a developmental anomaly. The benefits of making a diagnosis include the possibility of having more accurate discussions regarding prognosis, etiology, and recurrence risk. This is reviewed in more detail in Chapter 4 and throughout the rest of the book as it pertains to the diagnosis of a genetic syndrome or specific genetic disorder, such as hereditary deafness. However, these are the same goals for genomic medicine.

Genomic medicine is ". . . the routine use of genotypic analysis, usually in the form of DNA testing, to enhance the quality of medical care." This phrase was coined by the noted geneticist, Dr. Art Beaudet in his 1998 presidential address at the American Society of Human Genetics annual meeting (Beaudet, 1999), and is meant to describe the impact of the new wave of genetic information. Although the goal is to one day have genetic test results play an integral role in managing common diseases with very complex genetics, such as diabetes and psychiatric disease, genetic testing is already playing that role for several disorders. One example of that, hearing impairment, is discussed in detail in Chapter 9. Only a few years ago the genetic evaluation of hearing impairment was simple—identify whether the hearing impairment was part of a genetic syndrome. If it was not, there was little that could be done, even though it has long been known that a significant percentage of

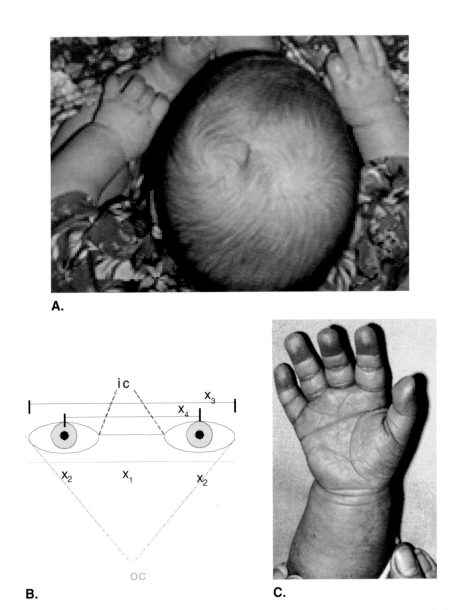

A.

B.   **C.**

FIGURE 1–3. A. The posterior hair whorl is formed secondary to brain growth during the second trimester. Most commonly there is a single hair whorl, slightly off-midline in the occipital parietal region. Many individuals have it in a different location, or have more than one, as is the case with this young child. By itself this has no clinical significance, however, if it is accompanied by microcephaly (small head size), developmental delay, and/or other neurologic findings, an aberrant hair whorl may indicate early abnormal brain growth. **B.** Normal eye spacing, where the space between the inner canthi (IC), x_1, is the same as a palpebral fissure lengths (eye openings), x_2. The IC is about one-third the length of the outer canthal distance (OC, x_3), and is 3 times the length of the IC. x_4 is the interpupilary distance. **C.** Palmar creases are an example of the subtle findings that a medical geneticist focuses on when evaluating a patient. (Courtesy of Raoul C. M. Hennekam, ICH, London.)

hearing impairment was due to genetic factors. Whatever counseling was provided was limited, and based on inexact empiric data. However, the discovery of the many hearing-related genes in the past decade has now enabled genetic testing for isolated hearing impairment and, therefore, more accurate counseling.

GENETICS MAY BE IMPORTANT, BUT WHY DO *I* HAVE TO KNOW THIS STUFF?

To this point, we have hopefully convinced you that genetics is a fascinating field, covering a vast array of information. That feature also makes genetics intimidating for many, as it combines clinical care with basic science concepts that are unfamiliar to most health care providers. This book aims to provide a window into the field for speech-language pathologists and audiologists that makes the field more understandable and, therefore, less intimidating. This is important for several reasons. Speech-language pathologists and audiologists are a primary contact for patients and their families. They will be asked questions about the child's problems, such as why it occurred. It is therefore important for them to be able to educate patients and parents about the process of a genetics evaluation, its benefits and limitations. In some cases, they may be the first to recognize that a patient would benefit from a genetics evaluation. Lastly, patients and parents may come to them and ask about a new genetic test that was discussed in the newspaper or that they heard about from a friend.

Genetics is not just in biomedical journals. Although it is true that medical journals feature research papers on genetics, genetics topics are also prominently featured in many lay publications, such as *U.S. News and World Report, Time, Newsweek,* and *Ladies Home Journal,* and local newspapers. Stories on genetics can be found on network news, local television and radio, and of course, the Internet. The bottom line is that you—and your patients and their families—will be hearing about genetics, whether it is the latest genetic finding, or a feature on a particular disorder. For example, the parents of a child with a speech delay will hear about the discovery of a gene involved in language development and will want to know about it, what it means, and how to get their child tested. These discussions are best left to the patients' physician, or even a geneticist or genetic counselor, but they often will be addressed first to the speech-language pathologist in an effort to get advice. So having some knowledge about this area is important.

A second more practical and perhaps more important reason is that you may be the first person to even consider the possibility of a genetic etiology for the child's problems. Consider the following two cases.

Case 1

A 3-year-old child is referred for a speech evaluation by his primary care physician. In the course of your evaluation you learn that the child had a congenital heart defect that was repaired in the newborn period. The child's facial appearance is not strikingly abnormal, but distinctive, different from that of his parents. Although you cannot place an exact name of diagnosis, you are suspicious that this child has a genetic syndrome. When you ask, the parents reply that they have never been seen by a geneticist before. They then ask why you asked about a geneticist.

Discussing with parents the possibility that their child has a genetic syndrome can be very difficult. However, it is important to do so, for if the child does indeed have a syndrome, it will greatly impact the child's current evaluation and treatment as well as future medical management plans. Although there is no "right" way to address this concern, it is typically best to focus the discussion on the medical benefits.

You respond to the parents saying that some cases of speech delay are caused by genetic factors. For that reason a genetic evaluation is often done to investigate this possibility.

Case 2

You are seeing a 3-year-old child for follow-up hearing testing. He was identified as hearing impaired when he failed his newborn hearing screen as well as repeat audiologic testing. The child is otherwise well, and there is no family history of hearing problems. His mother tells you that she and her husband are considering having another child, but are very concerned that the new child will also be hearing impaired. She asks you how likely is it that a subsequent child will have hearing impairment?

Obviously, this is a question that cannot be answered without more information. First it must be determined if the hearing impairment is isolated or part of a genetic syndrome. For isolated hearing impairment, many people think that because, there is no family history that the hearing impairment is not genetic. That is not accurate. About 50% of all hearing impairment is due to purely genetic factors, and most occurs without a family history. The possibility that the hearing impairment is genetic is also evident in the fact that normal-hearing, healthy parents of a hearing-impaired child have a significantly elevated risk for having a second hearing-impaired child, approximately 1 in 6.

The recent explosion of our understanding of the genetic basis of hearing has led to the creation of genetic tests, which can further refine these risks. In people of northern European descent, for example, there is approximately a 30% likelihood that the child's hearing impairment is due to a connexin 26 gene mutation. If positive, this means that the parents have a 1 in 4 risk of having a hearing impaired child with each future pregnancy. If negative, that risk is reduced only to 1 in 7, reflecting the fact that hearing impairment is genetically heterogeneous, so it is possible that other genes may underlie the child's hearing impairment.

Confusing? It is certainly a great deal of information. These topics are covered in more detail throughout the book, but it should be evident that answering this question requires a complete evaluation, genetic testing, and counseling. Although this is most likely something that is beyond what can happen during a brief follow-up visit, a proper referral to a geneticist can be made. The parents can be educated as to the need for an evaluation by a geneticist, what it entails, and what questions can, and cannot, be answered.

In short, that is the purpose of this book. We do not hope to make the reader into a geneticist—as discussed in Chapter 2, that would require several years of specialty training. Rather, the goal is to educate the reader as to what a medical genetics evaluation is, its benefits and limitations, and to remove some of the mystery behind this fast-moving and often-confusing field.

REFERENCE

Beaudet, A. (1999). Presidential address to the American Society of Human Genetics. *American Journal of Human Genetics*, 64, 1–13.

RECOMMENDED READING

Harper, P. S. (2004). *Landmarks in medical genetics.* Boston: Oxford University Press.

Childs, B. (2007). Medicine in a genetics context. In D. L. Rimoin, J. M. Connor, R. E. Pyeritz, & B. R. Korf (Eds.), *Emery & Rimoin's principles and practice of medical genetics* (5th ed.). St. Louis, MO: Elsevier.

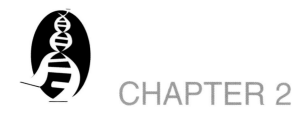

CHAPTER 2

Genetics Professionals:
An Overview

A confusing aspect of medical genetics is that so many different professionals are involved in patient care. Some are physicians; others are Ph.D.s. Many are master's-level genetic counselors or nurses with specialty training in genetics. Furthermore, most genetics centers are part of academic medical teaching institutions, so trainees of different levels are also common. In this chapter we review this "cast of characters," discussing their training and their respective roles in clinical care.

PHYSICIAN GENETICISTS

Many physicians from different specialties are experts in diseases that have a genetic basis. Examples include otolaryngologists whose expertise is hearing impairment, and plastic surgeons, whose focus is on congenital craniofacial anomalies. Although these individuals have an in-depth knowledge of the genetic basis of these specific disorders, they are not formally trained as geneticists. Just as otolaryngologists are doctors whose focus is on diseases of the head and neck and ears, a geneticist specializes in congenital disorders and diseases caused by genetic alterations. Traditionally, this has meant rare and primarily pediatric-age disorders, such as cleft palate and Down syndrome. Therefore, most geneticists have been pediatricians. With the recent explosion of genetic research, the number and scope of diseases that are considered "genetic" has greatly increased, and with it the role of the geneticist. Armed with a new array of tests, geneticists now have an expanded role, evaluating patients with disorders such as deafness, cancer, and heart failure. And as research continues to expand the number of diseases that are considered genetic will only increase.

Medical (or clinical) geneticists are physicians who have chosen genetics as their specialty. Nearly every clinical geneticist is also trained and certified in another specialty, most commonly Pediatrics, but geneticists also come from Obstetrics, Internal Medicine, and even Pathology training. Until the mid-1990s, medical genetics training was considered a "fellowship," meaning it was a subspecialty of one of these other disciplines. However, in 1993 Medical Genetics was recognized as the 23rd, and to date most recent medical specialty by the American Board of Medical Specialties (see Professional Organizations in Medical Genetics), achieving the same stature as other specialties such as Orthopedic Surgery or Psychiatry. Reflecting the fact that it is an independent specialty, physician trainees in Medical Genetics are now called residents.

There are several training tracks that one can take to become a medical geneticist. All begin with completing medical school. There are individuals, many very accomplished, who were trained many years ago who practice medical genetics but are not medical doctors; they hold either a Ph.D. or a D.D.S. (dental) degree. Today, it is required that all medical geneticists be medical doctors, although many also possess a Ph.D. as well. Furthermore, many geneticists who direct clinical genetics laboratories are Ph.D.s.

A genetics residency is 2 years in duration. To be eligible, one must have also completed at least 2 years in a primary care residency, such as Pediatrics or Internal Medicine, although many will complete 3 years so that they are board eligible. Compared to other specialties, there are very few genetics residency training programs in the United States. In early 2006 there were 46 programs listed, with a total of 77 filled training positions (http://www.acme.org/adspublic/reports/accredited_programs.asp).

There are three other training tracks for physicians to become a geneticist. Two of these are combined residency training programs with Pediatrics and Internal Medicine. Each is a 5-year program in which the resident alternates between Medical Genetics and Pediatrics (or Internal Medicine), and at the conclusion, residents are board eligible in both specialties (Medical Genetics and Pediatrics or Internal Medicine). Individuals enter these programs immediately after completing medical school. The other track is a combined fellowship in Maternal Fetal Medicine and residency in Medical Genetics. This program is a 4-year program in which the resident/fellow alternates between Medical Genetics and high-risk obstetrics. Individuals enter this program after completing a 4-year residency in Obstetrics and Gynecology. At the conclusion, the resident/fellow is board eligible in the specialties of Medical Genetics, Obstetrics and Gynecology, and Maternal Fetal Medicine.

As mentioned previously in this chapter, there are many areas of specialization within medical genetics. As with any specialty, geneticists are trained in each area, but typically will choose to focus their efforts in one.

> ### *Professional Organizations in Medical Genetics*
>
> **American Board of Medical Genetics** (ABMG) (http://genetics.faseb.org/genetics/abmg) is the primary body that certifies doctoral level medical genetics professionals (clinical geneticists, molecular geneticists, cytogeneticists, and biochemical geneticists). ABMG also accredits fellowships in cytogenetics, molecular genetics, and biochemical genetics. The ABMG is a member of the American Board of Medical Specialties,
>
> **American Society of Human Genetics** (ASHG) (http://genetics.faseb.org/genetics) is the oldest professional society for human geneticists, founded in 1948. The ASHG includes in its membership not only medical geneticists but also human genetics researchers. Like the ACMG, the ASHG also has important educational and public policy missions aimed to promote a greater understanding of genetics among the medical community and lay public.
>
> **American College of Medical Genetics** (http://www.acgme.net) is focused on the clinical application of genetics, including both laboratory practice as well as medical genetics care. Although it has no formal role in board certification, it does issue policy statements and practice guidelines on issues concerning the practice of medical genetics.
>
> **Accreditation Council on Graduate Medical Education** (http://www.acme.org) is the body that accredits postgraduate medical education programs (e.g., residencies and fellowships) for nearly all medical specialties in the United States. Each specialty has a residency review committee that periodically reviews each program. This is done to ensure that medical training is carried out at a uniformly high level in accordance with the guidelines set forth by the specialties governing body.
>
> **American Board of Genetic Counseling** (http://www.abgc.net) is the body that certifies genetic counselors and accredits genetic counseling training programs. It is an independent from the other groups listed.
>
> **National Society of Genetic Counselors** (http://www.NSGC.org) is the professional society for genetic counselors.

Dysmorphology

Dysmorphology is a term often used as a substitute for Pediatric Genetics, but it is its own separate area. It is the discipline that most doctors attribute to medical genetics. Dysmorphology, which is discussed in more detail in Chapters 4 and 5, is the study of abnormal form, but it has come to reflect the diagnosis and management of patients with a genetic syndrome. Although most patients are children, they may be of any age, including adults and even fetuses. The typical patient has one or more anomalies, such as mental retardation, hearing impairment, congenital heart defects, or other physical differences. Often patients will have a facial appearance that is unusual or is different than what would be expected for the family (unless one parent has the same genetic syndrome). The evaluation carried out by dysmorphologists (discussed in more detail in Chapter 4) includes a physical examination that looks at subtle physical differences that are seldom looked for by other physicians, such as eye spacing, creases on the palm, and hair pattern. These evaluations are often supplemented by laboratory testing, such as cytogenetic analysis and molecular genetic testing (discussed in more detail in Chapter 6). Finally, these evaluations typically include genetic counseling to summarize the impressions and results of the evaluation (discussed in more detail in Chapter 8).

Biochemical Genetics (Metabolism)

Similar to dysmorphology, biochemical genetics is a discipline primarily of pediatric-age patients. In contrast, however, these patients typically do not have physical anomalies—they are normal in their physical appearance. Instead, these patients have a defect in a metabolic pathway. These are referred to as inborn errors of metabolism (IEM). Some of the better known examples are phenlyketonuria, tyrosinemia, and maple syrup urine disease (MSUD). In these diseases, children are missing an enzyme that is involved in the synthesis or breakdown of an element that is important to the body's well-being. In the case of MSUD, certain amino acids (leucine, isoleucine, and valine, the so-called branch chain amino acids) cannot be broken down and recycled. And, like a road that is blocked due to construction or an accident, a buildup occurs. In some cases, the excessive precursors are shuttled to alternate pathways, leading to the formation of abnormal metabolites. Serious illness results due to a deficiency of the normal product of the blocked pathway, such as the case for disorders of energy metabolism (the ability to make energy-rich compounds like ATP), or the toxicity of the substrates and byproducts caused by the blockage. Management focuses on dietary manipulation to by-pass the blocked step in metabolism, and providing medical support when a decompensation occurs. These arise when children with IEM become catabolic, breaking down their own energy stores during times of stress (e.g., illness). This causes a sudden increase in toxic byproducts, leading to neurologic and other abnormalities.

Prenatal Genetics

This is the area of genetics with which lay people are most familiar, as many will see a genetic counselor or medical geneticist during a pregnancy. The focus of prenatal genetics is on screening and risk assessment to educate pregnant patients or those who are planning a pregnancy about their risk to have a baby with a medical problem. If screening tests have identified a problem, or raised the chance of a problem, further diagnostic testing can be recommended, such as chorionic villus sampling or amniocentesis (procedures by which a fetal chromosome analysis and DNA testing can be performed).

Prenatal genetics is important, as birth defects and genetic disease are, unfortunately, common. Even with no family history, about 1 to 3% of all babies are born with a birth defect or genetic disorder. The presence of a family history of a particular problem obviously raises that risk even further. Other things that raise the risk include advanced maternal age (over age 35 at the time of delivery); certain maternal health problems, such as insulin-dependent diabetes; and abnormalities found through routine prenatal tests, such as ultrasound or maternal serum screening. These are all addressed in the course of a prenatal genetics evaluation.

Cancer Genetics

With their discovery in the past decade, testing for cancer susceptibility genes has become a major component in the evaluation of patients with certain types of cancer, and/or those with a strong family history of cancer, even if the patient does not have a personal history of cancer. Breast, ovarian, and colon cancer have received the most attention, but genetic testing is also beneficial for other types of cancer, such as medullary thyroid cancer, melanoma, and retinoblastoma. Due to the complexities surrounding genetic testing (see Chapter 7 on Ethical Issues in Genetic Testing), many physicians treating these patients involve geneticists and/or genetic counselors in the testing process. As such, cancer genetics has emerged as a specialized discipline within medical genetics.

Adult Genetics

Adult genetics is an area of genetics that is still in its earliest stages of growth. It encompasses three different types of diseases. The first group are patients with pediatric genetic diseases who have gown to adulthood, such as adults with Down Syndrome or maple syrup urine disease. The second group is comprised of diseases, most of them relatively rare, that have a clear genetic basis but become evident only in adulthood, such as Marfan syndrome and Hemochromatosis. The third group includes diseases that are more common, and a subset of which are seen in families. The cancer genes discussed above are examples, but other diseases have followed a similar pattern with the genes being found in a subset of cases. Examples include hypertrophic cardiomyopathy and the polycystic kidney diseases. Identifying these genes has led to genetic testing for some of these, presenting opportunities for counseling families as well as improved medical management. Finally, the area that has received the greatest attention recently, especially in the popular press, is that of common diseases. Most common diseases, such as diabetes, stroke, and hypertension, have well-recognized genetic underpinnings. However, for each it is not a mutation in one gene that causes these diseases, but rather it is minor genetic variances (called polymorphisms) in many, perhaps dozens or more, genes that interact with environmental factors to produce the disease. Variations in these genes play an important but incomplete role. It is anticipated that identifying these genes and understanding their role(s) will lead to better treatments, and even cures, that are individualized to a specific patient. Take for example two patients with hypertension. Today, they would likely be treated with the same medication regimen. However, in the near future, genetic testing will be used to identify the underlying cause of each patient's hypertension. Testing may show that patient 1 has a different genetic profile than patient 2. With this insight, each patient can be treated with medications designed to address the underlying cause of the hypertension, which may be quite different. To achieve such personalized medical care (treatments based on a person's genotype) will require complex genetic testing, the ability to test a large number of genes simultaneously. Such technology is on the horizon, and with it comes potentially difficult legal, ethical, and societal issues. Although they cannot see each patient for testing for hypertension, it is expected that medical geneticists will be at the forefront of this emerging technology, providing guidance to their colleagues, and being involved in the most complicated or unusual cases.

OTHER GENETICS PROFESSIONALS

Medical geneticists are not the only genetics professionals involved in patient care. Other important personnel include genetic counselors, medical genetics residents, and laboratory geneticists. Furthermore, medical students and residents from other specialties often spend an elective month with the genetics service.

Laboratory Geneticists

Laboratory geneticists are Ph.D. or M.D. level professionals who carry out clinical genetic testing, usually as the director or assistant director of a laboratory. Some may also be involved in research, but that is separate from running a clinical laboratory. A clinical laboratory has a much different mission than a research laboratory, with safety measures regarding patient samples and protection of patient information held to a different regulatory standard than what is in place for research laboratories.

There are three main types of genetic testing labs—cytogenetics, molecular genetics, and biochemical genetics. Each type of testing is covered in more detail in Chapter 6. For each, a laboratory director (or assistant director) functions to supervise the overall activity of the lab, review and interpret each test, generate a report, and often communicate directly with the clinician who referred the patient for testing, especially in the case of positive results. Training to be a laboratory geneticist involves a separate track than what was described for a medical geneticist and is administered by a different supervisory body, the American Board of Medical Genetics (ABMG). The ABMG is also the governing body that administers the board certification test for both clinical laboratory geneticists as well as clinical geneticists and, in part, genetic counselors (see Professional Organizations in Medical Genetics).

Training for individuals with a Ph.D. involves 2 years of postgraduate clinical laboratory work in an accredited training program; for those with a medical degree, eligibility for board certification as a laboratory geneticist requires one additional year after the 2-year medical genetics residency.

Genetic Counselors

Genetic counselors are health professionals with specialized graduate degrees and experience in areas of medical genetics and counseling. They work as part of a genetics team to provide information and support to patients and their families. Through this process they gather information and investigate the problem present in the family to aid in establishing a diagnosis, while also working to communicate this information to the family and address concerns such as recurrence risks, support available at the community and state levels, and implications of this diagnosis for the individual and family unit. The process of genetic counseling is discussed in more detail in Chapter 8. Although genetic counselors provide genetic counseling, any health care provider can provide genetic counseling if he or she is knowledgeable of the topic, and has the necessary communication skills that genetic counselors learn in their training.

Genetic counselors are trained through a 2-year master's level program that focuses on medical genetics as well as counseling and interpersonal skills. At present, 27 accredited genetic counseling training programs are accredited by the American Board of Genetic Counseling (see http://www.abgc.net).

At the completion of their education, they are eligible to take a certification examination that is, in part, identical to that taken by clinical geneticists and clinical laboratory geneticists. Genetic counselors may work with a medical geneticist, assisting in their genetic evaluations, although others may work independently, or with limited involvement with a medical geneticist or other health care provider, in areas such as prenatal or cancer genetics. Regardless of the setting, counselors offer families information regarding their risk and options for testing, and assist in interpreting test results. Often counselors work in more than one area of practice, and their role may also include working in an administrative capacity or with research-related activities. In addition to providing these services and acting as advocates for their patients, genetic counselors facilitate referrals for their patients to other specialists or services, assist in navigating insurance issues, and act as educators to the public and other health care professionals regarding genetics.

Genetics Residents

Genetics residents were discussed previously in great detail with respect to their training and background. However, it is important to recognize that, although most medical genetics centers are based in academic medical centers and teaching hospitals, only a small percentage have their own medical genetics residency program. Therefore, most medical geneticists are not involved in medical genetics residency education, and most will not have a medical genetics resident with them. For the centers that do have such training programs, a medical genetics resident often is is the initial person involved in patient care. They report back to the attending medical geneticist, who supervises and guides the resident's activities.

Residents and Medical Students

Teaching is a major activity for most medical geneticists, as they typically are housed in major medical centers that have active medical schools and residency programs. Beyond teaching genetics residents, medical geneticists actively participate in teaching residents in other disciplines, such as Pediatrics, Internal Medicine, and Obstetrics and Gynecology, as well as medical students. This can include formal didactic contact, such as lectures or case discussions, or informal teaching that takes place in the course of discussing a particular patient. Furthermore, many residents and students spend time on the genetics service on a genetics elective rotation during their medical school education or residency training. For this reason it is common to see residents and students as part of the genetics team.

RECOMMENDED READING

Korf, B. R. (2005). Genetics in the genomic era. *Current Opinion in Pediatrics, 17,* 747–750.

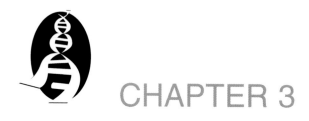

CHAPTER 3

Genetic Inheritance: Mendelian, Non-Mendelian, and Multifactorial

PEDIGREE NOTATION

Taking a detailed family history is important when evaluating a patient with a suspected genetically determined disease. It is best to develop a consistent and systematic manner, asking questions in a routine order so as not to forget any important points. Although the questions on the indication for referral (e.g., for a hearing impaired child, asking if anyone else in the family has a hearing impairment) should, of course, be included, more general information should also be sought, as it may prove to be important in reaching a genetic diagnosis. For example, in the hearing impaired child, a family history of early onset arthritis would suggest the diagnosis of Stickler syndrome. How such associated findings can lead to the diagnosis of a genetic syndrome is covered more completely in Chapter 4.

Recording the family history is best done by using standardized pedigree notation, as is illustrated in Figure 3–1. By using this system, the information is depicted in a simple yet detailed manner, permitting easy interpretation of the information. How that information is interpreted is the subject of this chapter.

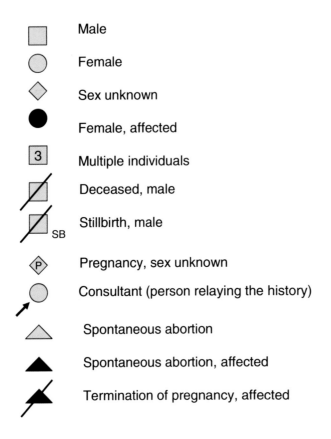

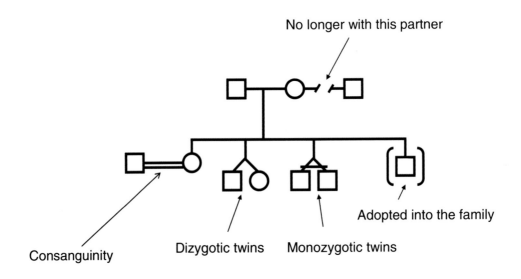

FIGURE 3–1. Symbols commonly used in pedigree notation.

GENETIC INHERITANCE

There are many different forms of genetic inheritance. In some cases, having a genetic change is all that is needed for an individual to express a particular **phenotype** (Table 3-1). Sometimes, the trait or disease can be traced (inherited) within a family using **pedigree notation**. There are three forms of this type of genetic inheritance: **autosomal dominant, autosomal recessive,**

TABLE 3–1. Definition of Commonly Encountered Genetics Terms

Gene: The basic unit of heredity, consisting of a DNA segment arranged in a linear manner along a chromosome. A gene codes for a specific protein

Genotype: The genetic constitution of an organism or cell; also refers to the specific set of alleles inherited at a locus

Allele: One version of a gene at a given location (locus) along a chromosome

Locus: The physical site or location of a specific gene on a chromosome

Phenotype: The observable physical, biochemical, or behavioral characteristics of the expression of a gene; the clinical presentation of an individual with a particular genotype

Heterozygote: An individual who has two different alleles at a particular locus, one on each chromosome of a pair; one allele is usually normal and the other abnormal

Mutation: Any alteration in a gene from its natural state; may be disease-causing or a benign, normal variant

Allelic variant of unknown significance: An alteration in the normal sequence of a gene, the significance of which is unclear until further study of the genotype and corresponding phenotype in a sufficiently large population; complete gene sequencing often identifies numerous (sometimes hundreds) allelic variants for a given gene

Benign variant: (synonym: polymorphism) An alteration in a gene distinct from the normal, wild-type allele that does not appear to have a deleterious effect

Locus heterogeneity: The situation in which mutations in genes at different chromosomal loci cause the same phenotype

Variable expressivity: Variation in clinical features (type and severity) of a genetic disorder between affected individuals, even within the same family

Penetrance: The proportion of individuals with a mutation causing a particular disorder who exhibit clinical symptoms of that disorder; most often refers to autosomal dominant conditions

Allelic heterogeneity: (synonym: molecular heterogeneity) Different mutations in the same gene at the same chromosomal locus that cause a single phenotype

Source: Adapted from: GeneTests [http://www.geneclinics.org]. Accessed August, 2005.

and **X-linked**. They are termed **Mendelian** inheritance, after a 19th century Austrian monk, Gregor Mendel. From his experiments on how certain traits in garden peas were passed down came Mendel's laws of inheritance, which still form the foundation of our understanding of genetic transmission today.

More than 6000 different diseases inherited in this manner are listed in OMIM (http://www.ncbi.nlm.nih.gov/). However, there are many more diseases that do not follow a classic inheritance pattern, in which the presence of the abnormal gene is by itself sufficient to cause the disease. These are called **complex genetic traits.** For these, the presence of separate "modifier" genes or environmental factors determines if the particular disease will emerge in an individual. The remainder of this chapter reviews the various forms of genetic inheritance, using commonly encountered diseases as examples.

MENDELIAN INHERITANCE

Autosomal Dominant Inheritance

To understand autosomal dominant inheritance, it is necessary to recall that our genes exist on chromosomes. These are found in 23 pairs, numbered 1 (the largest) through 22 (the smallest), with the last pair being the two sex chromosomes, X and Y—women have 2 Xs, whereas men have an X and a Y. Numbers 1 through 22 are called the **autosomes**. For an autosomal dominant disorder, only one gene of the pair is changed, but the effect of the changed gene dominates the normal gene and is sufficient to cause the abnormal phenotype (Figure 3-2).

There are several ways that a single changed gene can result in an abnormal phenotype. The gene can lose its ability to produce a protein (partially or completely), or produce a protein that has diminished or absent function, (so-called hypomorphic, or amorphic mutations, respectively); the gene prod-

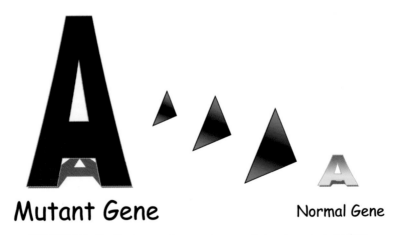

Mutant Gene   Normal Gene

FIGURE 3–2. Cartoon of an autosomal dominant mutation.

uct's function may become too strong (hypermorphic); or even take on a new deleterious function, either by its own toxic action (neomorphic), or in interacting with normal proteins (protein suicide).

There are several characteristics of autosomal dominant inheritance. These are demonstrated in the sample autosomal dominant pedigree in Figure 3–3, and include:

1. Vertical, or parent to child, transmission. This is illustrated by individual I.1 passing on the changed gene to II.2 and II.5.

2. Fifty percent (1/2) recurrence risk for affected individuals for *each* pregnancy. Although this means *on average*, half of an affected person's offspring will inherit the changed gene and the trait, it is important to remember that there is a 50% chance *with each pregnancy*.

3. Unaffected individuals do not pass on the trait. This is because, if one does not inherit the changed gene and the trait, it cannot be passed on. This assumes that the genetic mutation is *completely penetrant*, a concept that is discussed in more detail below.

4. Males and females are equally likely to be affected, and are affected in the same way.

5. Although not a "rule" per se, the finding of male-to-male transmission essentially confirms that the condition is inherited as an autosomal dominant trait. Male-to-male inheritance is also seen with Y-linked inheritance, which is discussed in more detail below. But since there are very few Y-linked traits compared to autosomal dominant traits, it is safe to assume male-to-male inheritance indicates autosomal dominant inheritance. This is seen in Figure 3–3 where father I.1 passed on the trait to his son, II.5, and II.5 passed it on to III.7.

Many autosomal dorminant diseases and pedigrees seem not to follow these rules. These exceptions serve to illustrate several important principals of genetic inheritance.

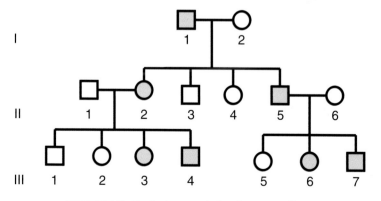

FIGURE 3–3. Autosomal dominant pedigree.

New Mutation

Although autosomal dominant diseases occur in families, in many instances the genetic change first occurred in the individual that you are seeing. In such cases, both parents are unaffected, and there is no family history. For example, the child in Figure 11–11 has Achondroplasia, the most common genetic form of dwarfism. It is caused by a specific change in a gene called *fibroblast growth factor receptor 3* (*FGFR3*). Although affected individuals can pass on the genetic change, and hence the condition, to their offspring according to the rules of autosomal dominant inheritance, as described above, about 80% of cases occur with no family history. The genetic change occurred in the egg or sperm that formed the child, and is classified as a "new mutation." In these cases it can be difficult to differentiate a "new dominant" mutation from an autosomal recessive or X-linked disorder (see below).

For some autosomal dominant disorders, such as lethal disorders, all cases represent new mutations. One such example is Thanatophoric dysplasia, which is a lethal skeletal disorder caused by different mutations in FGFR3.

Variable Expression

Expression refers to the severity that a genetic alteration affects an individual. Not all individuals with the same autosomal dominant genetic change manifest a genetic condition the same way. One example is Stickler syndrome, a genetically determined disorder characterized by vision abnormalities (high myopia and retinal detachment); early onset osteoarthritis; hearing loss; and facial differences that can include cleft palate and Pierre Robin sequence (see Chapter 10) At the most severe end of the spectrum, individuals have most or all of these complications. However, most are more mildly affected, with few or even just one finding to suggest the presence of the mutant gene. This is referred to as *variable expression*. In taking a family history an individual who has the condition may be missed because their findings are milder or, less commonly more severe, than your patient. In taking a family history, such affected individuals may not be recognized as being in the spectrum of the same disorder.

Incomplete Penetrance

Some autosomal dominant disorders appear to skip a generation (Figure 3–4). When an individual carries a genetic mutation but does not manifest any clinical findings it is termed "incomplete penetrance," and the disorder is classified as being "incompletely penetrant." For such disorders, the penetrance can be calculated easily, as the percentage of gene carriers who manifest some aspect of the associated phenotype divided by the number of mutation carriers.

To use an analogy, penetrance is like an on/off light switch—the light is either on or off. Similarly, the condition is either penetrant or not: it either shows some phenotypic finding or it does not. In contrast, *expressivity* is like a dimmer switch, in which the light is on and can be gradually adjusted to be either very bright or dim (Figure 3-5).

There are many reasons that a condition exhibits reduced penetrance. Some gene mutations require the presence of other factors to appear, such as environmental agents or modifier genes. For example, the mitochondrial mutation in the mitochondrial genome, A1555G, will cause early-onset hearing loss if an individual is exposed to an aminoglycoside antibiotic. If a person who carries this mutation is never given this type of antibiotic, they will experience hearing loss at a later age, if at all.

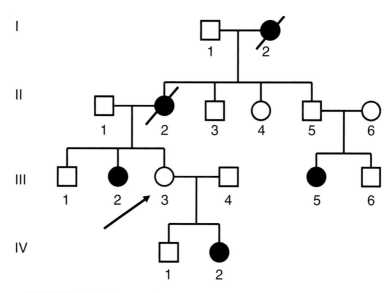

FIGURE 3–4. Incomplete penetrance: III.3 is nonpenetrant.

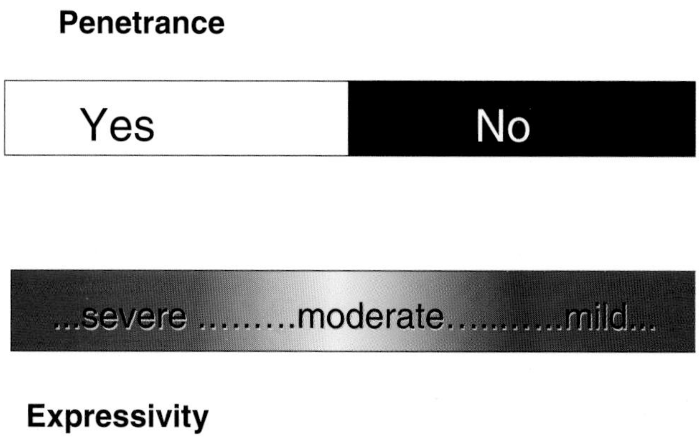

Penetrance

Yes	No

...severe ....moderate...........mild...

Expressivity

FIGURE 3–5. Cartoon depictions of the concepts of penetrance (*black or white, yes or no*) and expressivity (*various shades of gray*).

Sex, age, and chance can also influence penetrance. Mutations in genes associated with breast and ovarian cancer are more likely to manifest in woman simply due to male versus female anatomy. Therefore, a male with a BRCA1 mutation would be determined to be nonpenetrant, as is the case for II.5 in Figure 3-5. For a completely penetrant genetic disorder like Huntington disease, essentially 100% of mutation carriers will develop neurological signs. However, the risk of developing symptoms increases with age, so that a healthy young woman who carries a Huntington disease associated mutation would be called nonpenetrant, although she will almost certainly develop the disease at some point in her life and be penetrant. Finally, for some diseases such as BRCA1/2 associated breast and ovarian cancer, a subset of gene mutation carriers simply will not develop disease.

Germline Mosaicism

Some genetic mutations occur not in the egg or sperm that forms a child, but rather in a cell in the developing embryo. Such events are referred to as **somatic mutations**. The phenotype caused by a somatic mutation can be very varied, but is usually milder than if all cells contained the genetic mutation, so-called **germline mutations**. In some cases, the somatic mutation occurs in cells that populate the germline and produce eggs or sperm. Although these individual may have few if any manifestations of the disorder, they will produce many eggs or sperm that carry the mutation, resulting in unaffected parents having more than one child with an autosomal dominant genetic disorder. In this way, it can mimic autosomal recessive inheritance.

Autosomal Recessive Inheritance

In contrast to autosomal dominant inheritance, in which only one of the pair of a specific gene is altered, autosomal recessive inheritance requires mutations in both copies of the gene. Well known examples of autosomal recessive diseases include cystic fibrosis, sickle cell disease, and connexin 26-related hearing impairment. Autosomal recessive pedigrees also have their own characteristics (Figure 3-6). These include:

1. Horizontal transmission, the observation of multiple affected members in the same generation, but no affected family members in other generations.

2. Recurrence risk of 25% for parents with a previous child with an autosomal recessive disease. This is because both parents are assumed to be carriers. Although theoretically possible, it is extremely unlikely for only one parent to be a carrier and the mutation on the other chromosome to have arisen as a new event. When assessing recurrence risk and carrier status, it is most easy to use a Punnet square (Figure 3-7).

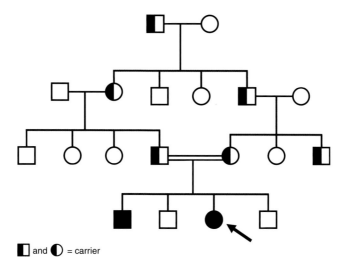

FIGURE 3–6. Autosomal recessive pedigree.

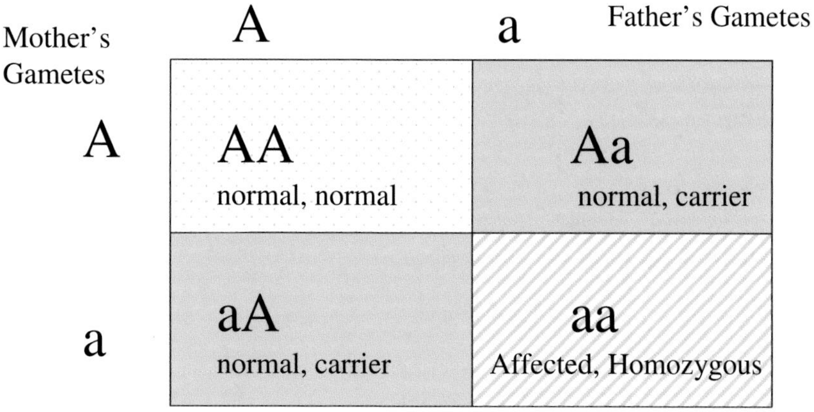

Mother's Gametes	A	a — Father's Gametes
A	AA normal, normal	Aa normal, carrier
a	aA normal, carrier	aa Affected, Homozygous

FIGURE 3–7. Punnet square for an autosomal recessive trait.

3. Males and females equally affected, unless the specific condition has different expression in males and females (see discussion of BRCA1 above).

4. Consanguinity (a close biological relationship between parents, such as first cousins) can be seen with autosomal recessive disorders, especially if it is a very rare disorder. This reflects the fact that related individuals share a greater proportion of their genes, including carrying recessive mutations.

   While consanguinity is meant to refer to a close biological relationship between parents, the notion of shared ancestry and a limited gene pool is also seen in the concept of **Founder Effect**. This refers to the recognition that many autosomal recessive genetic diseases occur more commonly in certain ethnically defined groups. Tay Sachs disease is one such example. This lethal neurodegenerative disease is very rare among the general population, but far more common among Ashkenazi Jews, who have a carrier rate for TSD of 1 in 31.

Pseudodominant Inheritance

Pseudodominant inheritance refers to the observation of parent-to-child transmission of a known autosomal recessive trait (Figure 3–8). This gives the appearance of autosomal dominant transmission, but it is known that the disease is autosomal recessive. This occurs in conditions that are relatively mild and compatible with reproduction that have a high carrier frequency in a population, either by a founder effect (see above), consanguinity, or a selection bias. An example is deafness related to *GJβ2* mutations. *GJβ2* is the gene for Connexin 26, and mutations in this gene are the most common genetic form of deafness, causing 30% sporadic (no family history) congenital deafness, and 55% when the family history suggests autosomal recessive inheritance in certain populations. The carrier rate for a *GJβ2* mutation is about 1 in 31 for individuals of Northern European descent. However, the risk that a *GJβ2* homozygote would have children with a *GJβ2* carrier is even greater than what the carrier rate would indicate. Due to shared culture and lifestyles, a deaf person is more likely to have children with another deaf person, or at least a person familiar with deafness, such as the sibling of a deaf person. Similarly, the hearing sibling of a deaf person would be more open to marrying a

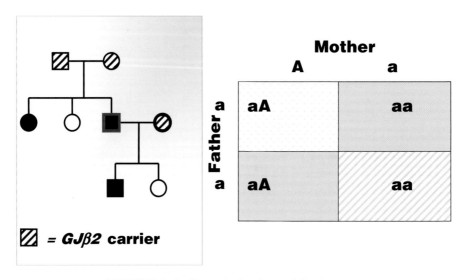

FIGURE 3–8. Pseudodominant inheritance.

deaf person due to their familiarity with sign language and the other aspects of being deaf. So as before, the likelihood that a *GJβ2* homozygote would meet a *GJβ2* carrier is even greater than what the carrier rate would indicate. Every pregnancy between a *GJβ2* homozygote and carrier would have a 1 in 2 chance of producing a deaf child, the same as what is seen with an autosomal dominant trait.

X-Linked Inheritance

X-linked inheritance is commonly divided in to X-linked recessive and X-linked dominant based on whether or not a carrier female manifests signs of the disease. If female carriers are normal, the disease is termed X-linked recessive; if they manifest some aspect of the disorder, it is X-linked dominant. Like autosomal dominant and autosomal recessive traits, pedigrees demonstrating X-linked inheritance have certain characteristics (Figure 3–9):

1. Males are more often and more severely affected than females.

2. Female carriers are generally healthy, or at least more mildly affected than males with the X-linked genetic mutation.

3. Affected men will have only carrier daughters. They have no chance of having an affected son (remember, male-to-male transmission excludes X-linked inheritance, and is seen with autosomal dominant and Y-linked inheritance).

4. Carrier women will have a 25% risk for having an affected son, a 25% risk for carrier daughters, and a 50% chance of having a child that does not inherit the mutated X-linked gene (Figure 3–10).

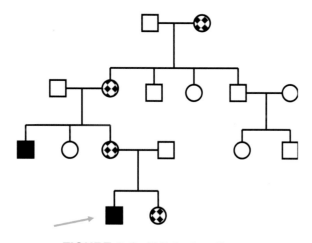

FIGURE 3–9. X-linked pedigree.

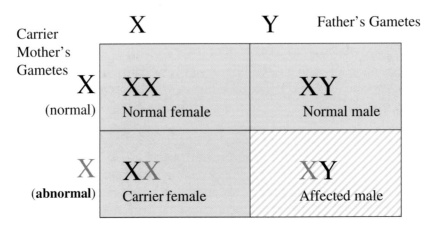

FIGURE 3–10. Punnet square for X-linked inheritance.

Although most X-linked diseases primarily affect males, there are several reasons that a female carrier may manifest the disease to the same extent as a male. One reason is due to abnormal *X-inactivation*. In females, one of the X-chromosomes becomes inactive early in the development of the embryo. There are many reasons, including random chance, that the X-chromosome that contains the *normal* X-linked gene is inactivated in the vast majority of cells (so-called skewed X-inactivation).

A female will manifest an X-linked disease if she is homozygous for the X-linked mutant gene. Such cases are rare, and usually involve relatively mild conditions that are fairly common, such as X-linked color blindness. In such cases, the affected daughter would be born to an affected male and carrier female.

Another reason for a female to manifest an X-linked disorder would be that the affected female has only one X chromosome. Examples include Turner syndrome (45,X), or a case of sex reversal, such as androgen insensitivity, in which an individual has a 46,XY chromosome complement but appears as a phenotypic female due to the absence of response to the normal effects of male hormones (androgens).

Y-Linked Inheritance

Pedigrees exhibiting Y-linked inheritance show *only* male-to-male transmission and only males are affected. However, few conditions produce such a pedigree. That is because the Y chromosome is the smallest human chromosome, containing the fewest genes, and most are related to male sex determination and reproduction. Mutations in these genes typically cause male infertility, and are, therefore, usually not passed down. However, with modern assisted reproduction techniques, many infertile males can now father children, so it is possible to pass on these Y-linked traits.

Digenic Inheritance

Digenic inheritance refers to the coinheritance of mutations in two different genes. Neither one by itself causes disease, but together they do. An example of this is Retinitis Pigmentosa (RP), a common genetic form of blindness that is very heterogeneous, with several autosomal dominant and autosomal recessive forms. Mutations in ROM1 and rhodopsin (Rho) each can cause autosomal recessive RP. Like any autosomal recessive disease, individuals who are carriers of either a Rho or ROM1 mutation are clinically normal. However, individuals who are double carriers—have one mutant RMO1 allele and one mutant RHO allele—develop RP just as they would had they been homozygous for mutations in either RHO or ROM1.

Digenic pedigrees (Figure 3–11) exhibit characteristics of both autosomal dominant (vertical transmission) and autosomal recessive inheritance (1 in 4 recurrence risk). Although there are only very few recognized digenically inherited disorders, that list is sure to grow in the future, and even include more complex situations with two, three, four, and more genes interacting to produce a specific disease.

Pseudogenetic Inheritance

Mutant genes are not the only cause for a disease to demonstrate familial transmission. Exposure to a teratogen, chance, and social and environmental factors all may cause familial clustering of a disease and thereby mimick genetic transmission. For example, a woman with phenylketonuria, a disorder in which affected people cannot break down certain amino acids, may have

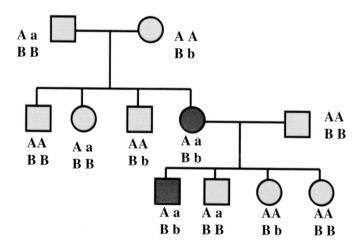

Genes A and B are unlinked, and therefore segregate independently.

FIGURE 3–11. Digenic pedigree.

multiple children with mental retardation. In this instance, the genetic disease is not the direct cause of the mental retardation in the offspring—they are each only a carrier for PKU. Rather, it is the toxic effect on the developing fetus of the byproducts from their mother's metabolic disease. Similarly, an alcoholic woman will have multiple children with fetal alcohol syndrome due to her use of alcohol during pregnancy, not due to genetic transmission.

Some familial clustering occurs simply because they have a high frequency in the general population. For example, a common disease like colon or breast cancer may occur in several members of a family due to the fact that these are common diseases. This is distinct from the familial clustering seen with a genetically determined cancer-predisposition syndrome, like that seen with mutations in BRCA1 or 2. Such families have earlier onset than typical sporadic breast cancer.

Familial clustering of a cancer may also be a clue to an environmental exposure. For example, exposure to excessive radiation or asbestos each can lead to familial clusterings of certain cancers as well as other medical problems.

Finally, social factors may also mimic genetic transmission of a disease. For example, obese parents are more likely to have overweight children. Although there may be genetic factors contributing, poor diet and exercise habits are also major contributors.

NONTRADITIONAL INHERITANCE

So far we have reviewed the classic forms of genetic transmission. Although each was different, with its own rules and characteristics, they shared several basic principles:

1. There are equal maternally derived and paternally derived contributions to an individual's genome (with the obvious exception of X- and Y-linked genes);

2. The maternal and paternal alleles of a gene are functionally equivalent;

3. Genetic mutations are static—the alteration in the gene does not change across generations. Although the phenotype may be different among members of a family due to variable expression or reduced penetrance, the actual alteration of the genetic sequence is identical between those individuals;

4. Two copies of autosomal genes are sufficient for health. In some cases one functional copy can suffice, as is seen in carriers of an autosomal recessive trait, but two normal copies are optimal.

In this last section, we described several forms of genetic inheritance that do not hold to these principles. Called either "nontraditional" or "non-Mendelian" forms of inheritance, these are relatively newly identified mechanisms for transmission of a genetic disease.

Mitochondrial Inheritance

An individual's mitochondrial genome is entirely derived from his or her mother. Mitochondrial in the sperm are located in the tail and do not typically enter the ovum after fertilization. Therefore, the father's mitochondrial genome is not passed down. Mitochondrial disorders exhibit "maternal" inheritance, that is, a woman with a mitochondrial genetic disorder will have only affected offspring, whereas an affected father will have no affected offspring (Figure 3–12). Although such an inheritance pattern can be explained by autosomal dominant of X-linked inheritance, it should strongly suggest a mitochondrial basis.

The mitochondria are the cell's suppliers of energy, so that the organs that are most affected by the presence of abnormal mitochondria are those that have the greatest energy requirements, such as the brain, muscles, sensory organs, and liver. Common signs and symptoms of mitochondrial disorders include developmental delay/mental retardation, seizures, cardiac dysfunction, decreased strength and tone, and hearing and vision problems. Examples include MELAS (myopathy, encephalopathy, lactic acidosis, and strokelike episodes), MERRF (myoclonic epilepsy associated with ragged-red fibers), and Kearns-Sayre syndrome (ophthalmoplegia, pigmentary retinopathy, and cardiomyopathy). However, mitochondrial diseases can be exceptionally variable in the clinical manifestations. This is due to unequal segregation of abnormal mutant mitochondria in daughter cells. This proportion is referred to as "heteroplasmy" and determines how severely a given organ is affected. For this reason, taking a careful pedigree is crucial because the phenotype can vary even within a family, and it is possible to overlook a mildly affected family member.

Finally, it is important to remember the distinction between a mitochondrial inheritance and a mitochondrial disease. Although all mitochondrial genes make proteins that are used by the mitochondrion to make ATP, these are only a small number of the proteins needed for this activity. The majority of these several dozen proteins are encoded by nuclear genes. That is why most mitochondrial diseases are inherited in an autosomal recessive manner.

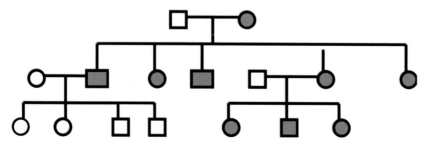

FIGURE 3–12. Maternal inheritance pedigree.

Triplet Repeat Disorders

Triplet repeat disorders represent a special type of Mendelian inheritance. They are distinguished by **genetic anticipation**, the observed trait that the condition worsens over generations, in severity and/or age of onset. Triplet repeat disorders include well-known disorders, like Fragile X syndrome, myotonic dystrophy, and Huntington disease, as well as over a dozen rare neurodegerative disorders, like Kennedy disease and Freidreich ataxia. Although each of these disorders is inherited in an X-linked, autosomal dominant, or autosomal recessive pattern, they each have unusual genetics characteristics that differentiate them from disorders with typical Mendelian inheritance patterns. This is because, unlike the types of mutations discussed elsewhere, triplet repeat mutations are not static; they change as they are passed down from parent to child.

Triplet repeat disorders are caused by expansion in the number of three-base pair repeats within a gene. For example, the Fragile X gene, FMR1, has between 5 and 50 CGG triplets in the normal state; for the myotonic dystrophy gene (myotonin protein kinase on chromosome 19q), the number of repeats is 5 to 40. However, an error in meiosis can result in a small expansion in that number. This is referred to as a "premutation." For Fragile X, that number is 50 to 200 repeats, for myotonic dystrophy it is 50 to 100. Individuals with a premutation are typically well, with few if any phenotypic findings.[1] However, these individuals are at risk for having the gene expand further in subsequent meiosis, crossing into the range of full mutation. For Fragile X, that boundary is above 200 repeats. With this number of repeats, the FMR1 gene becomes hypermethylated, and protein production is lost. The effect of the expansion is different in other genes. For Huntington disease the expansion causes the gene product to have a new, toxic effect on the neurons of the basal ganglia. For most triplet repeat disorders, there is a clinical correlation to the size of the expansion, with a greater expansion causing more severe and/or earlier age of onset for the disease. This is the molecular explanation for the clinical observation of genetic anticipation.

Genetic Imprinting

For most genes in the human genome, two active copies are considered normal, and these genes are function equivalent. This is one of the basic tenants of genetics. Although this is true for most genes, we now know that this is not true for all genes. However, for a small number, one of the pair is turned off, made transcriptionally silent. Called **genetic imprinting**, this is not due to

---

[1]Recent research on Fragile X premutation carriers has shown that they may manifest one of three distinct clinical disorders: mild cognitive and/or behavioral deficits on the fragile-X spectrum; premature ovarian failure; and a tremor/ataxia syndrome (Hagerman & Hagerman, 2004).

an alteration in the DNA sequence of the gene. Rather, it is hypermethylated, so-called "epigenetic modification." This process occurs in either the male or female germ line, depending on the specific gene. For some genes, only the maternally derived copy is active, whereas for others it is the paternal copy. Some of these genes are subjected to imprinting in one tissue but, in other parts of the body, there is bi-allelic (both copies) expression.

Imprinted genes are typically found in clusters scattered throughout the genome. Each cluster typically has an "imprinting center" that controls which genes are silenced. Interestingly, the genes within an imprinted region are not all imprinted in the same manner—for some the maternal copy is expressed, for others it is the paternal copy.

Imprinting disorders result from an imbalance of active copies of a given gene, which can occur for several reasons. This is illustrated in the best known example of imprinting disorders, Prader-Willi and Angelman syndromes. These are clinically very different disorders. Prader-Willi syndrome is characterized by moderate mental retardation with very specific behavior (bad temper, affinity for puzzles), short stature, hypogenetalism in males, and characteristic facies (Figure 3–13). Early in life these children are extremely hypotonic, but then later become hyperphagic, so that morbid obesity becomes a major problem. Recent studies have shown that behavioral modification and treatment with growth hormone can be beneficial to overall health. Clinically, this

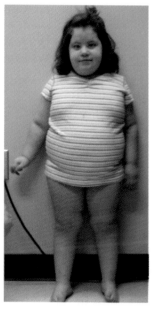

FIGURE 3–13. A 6-year-old girl with Prader-Willi syndrome. In addition to the obesity note the characteristic subtle physical findings: bitemporal narrowing, almond-shaped eyes that are slanting, and small hands and feet.

is in sharp contrast to Angelman syndrome, which is characterized by more severe mental retardation, seizures, ataxic gait, and absent speech. Individuals with Angelman syndrome manifest unexplained bouts of laughter, and have a marked affinity for water. They are not obese.

It was surprising, then, that these two very different syndromes were found to be caused by apparently identical cytogenetic deletions of chromosome 15q11-12. However, the deletion in Prader-Willi syndrome patients always was found to be on the paternally derived chromosome 15, while that seen with Angelman syndrome is on the maternal copy. We now know the specific gene for Angelman syndrome. Called UBE3A, the paternal copy is silenced. Mutations in the paternally derived copy of UBE3A have no effect, but those in the maternal UBE3A leave no functioning and result in Angelman syndrome.

There are other genetic mechanisms that can cause Prader-Willi and Angelman syndromes, as well as other imprinting disorders. One is uniparental disomy (UPD), the rare occurrence of a child inheriting both copies of a chromosome from the same parent. For example, inheriting both chromosome 15s from the mother will cause functionally the same as a deletion of the paternal 15q12, and will likewise result in Prader-Willi syndrome. About 30% of Prader-Willi syndrome is caused by paternal UPD15, whereas maternal UPD15 accounts for only 3% or Angelman syndrome. Mutations in UBE3 account for almost one third of Angelman syndrome cases, and can also result in familial transmission. Lastly, the rarest cause is a mutation in the imprinting center. This results in an inability to set the imprint. In a woman, for example, the inability to reset their father's chromosome 15 imprint will result in passing on no active copies of UBE3, and the child will have Angelman syndrome. It is another potential reason that one might see familial transmission of an imprinted disorder. By either mechanism, such pedigrees are very unusual, containing skipped generations with nonpenetrant gene carriers.

Besides 15q11-12, there are many other regions in the genome that are subjected to imprinting. These include the short arm of chromosome 11 (the genes for two imprinted disorders, Beckwith-Wiedemann syndrome and nesidioblastosis, map to this area); and the long arm of chromosome 7 (maternal uniparental disomy of 7q has been associated with some cases of idiopathic short stature and Russell Silver syndrome). As is the case for chromosome 15q11-12, the genes within a region are not imprinted in the same manner. For some the maternal copy may be expressed, whereas for others within the same region the paternally derived copies are expressed.

Other chromosomes, 2, 13, and 22 for example, do not seem to have any imprinted regions. Finally, although most imprinting disorders are sporadic (occur with no family history), there are rare cases of familial occurrence of an imprinting disorder. When these occur they manifest an unusual pedigree, with skipped generations and consistent (maternal or paternal) transmitting family members.

Multifactorial/Polygenic Inheritance

Not all congenital abnormalities are determined by a chromosomal abnormality or a single abnormal gene. Multifactorial inheritance refers to a disorder that is caused by a combination of genetic, environmental, and stochastic factors. Multifactorial traits are different from polygenic inheritance, which refers to disorders that result from the additive effects of multiple genes. Digenic inheritance (discussed above) is the simplest example of this form of inheritance.

Multifactorial conditions segregate within families, but do not exhibit a consistent or recognizable inheritance pattern. However, like other forms of genetic inheritance there are several characteristics for multifactorial inheritance. These include that the abnormality usually involves one organ system or related system; is concordant more often among monozygotic twins than dizygotic twins; the recurrence risk is greater if more than one offspring is affected (indicating a greater genetic contribution); the risk diminishes for more remote relatives; the more severely affected the proband the greater the recurrence risk; if the disorder is more frequent in one sex, the risk is greater for relatives of patients if the proband is of the less frequently affected sex (e.g., a girl with pyloric stenosis, which is fivefold more common in boys).

There are two types of multifactorial traits. The first type is termed quantitative. Such traits exhibit continuous variation, with normal defined by a statistical range, and outliers of that range, usually two standard deviations, considered abnormal. Intelligence, blood pressure, and height and head circumference are examples. For such characteristics, offspring tend to represent a modified average of their parents, with nutritional and environmental factors also playing an important role as well in the final result.

Other multifactorial traits can be more clearly distinguished between normal and abnormal. These are called qualitative traits, and examples include pyloric stenosis, neural tube defects, congenital heart defects, and cleft lip and cleft palate. Such traits follow a threshold model. Every individual has a certain level of genetic variation, some of which creates an increased susceptibility to a certain condition. Various liability factors (see Chapter 10, Figure 10–9) are additive, and if their sum exceeds a threshold, the trait will manifest. Such factors are both genetic and environmental. For example, an exposure to a teratogen such as dilantin or the rubella virus would move the threshold to the left of the normal distribution, raising the likelihood of developing a birth defect.

The balance between genetic and environmental factors is demonstrated by a neural tube defect. Genetic factors are implicated by the increased recurrence risk for parents of an affected child compared to the general population. However, this risk is 3%, less than what would be expected if the trait was caused by a single gene. Further emphasizing the role of nongenetic, environmental factors is that the recurrence risk can be lowered by up to 70% if the mother-to-be takes folic acid at 4 mg/day starting 3 months prior to conception. Only a few such genetic or environmental liability factors have been identified. One recent discovery was that a sequence variation in the *interferon regulatory factor 6* gene was associated with an increased risk for cleft lip and palate.

Many adult onset diseases are also multifactorial. Diabetes, coronary artery disease, and schizophrenia are a few examples where a great deal of research has taken place into the genetic factors that underlie these diseases. Such discoveries will aid not only in identifying individuals at increased risk so that they can take preventative measures, but also to provide insights into basic disease mechanism to assist in designing therapies.

REFERENCE

Hagerman, P. J., & Hagerman, R. S. (2004). The fragile X permutation: A maturing perspective. *American Journal of Human Genetics*, 74, 805–816.

RECOMMENDED READING

Harper, P. S. (2004). *Practical genetic counseling* (6th ed.). London: Hodder Arnold.

Korf, B. R. (2007). *Human genetics and genomics* (3rd ed.). Oxford, UK: Blackwell.

Nussbaum, R. L., McInnes, R. R., & Willard, H. F. (2001). *Thompson & Thompson genetics in medicine* (6th ed.). New York: W. B. Saunders.

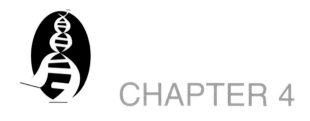

CHAPTER 4

The Evaluation of the Patient with a Congenital Anomaly

*T*he child with a congenital anomaly presents a special and difficult challenge to both the health care team and the child's family. Parents are often overwhelmed with medical concerns as well as complex emotions, and the child's health care providers are understandably focused on the health issues related to the anomaly. Immediate medical concerns include identifying the extent and etiology of the anomalies, potential for functional correction or cosmetic improvement, and possibility of associated developmental limitations or cognitive impairment. Although the psychosocial context will certainly vary, families commonly experience grieving over the loss of the expected "healthy" child, guilt for believing they contributed to the cause of the congenital anomalies in their child, difficulty bonding or feeling the expected joy at the birth of a child, financial concern related to expected surgeries or chronic medical management, and a wider concern for whether other family members may be at risk for similar problems. Ethical issues may arise, such as whether to proceed with chronic support or surgical intervention for a child with a poor prognosis. Lastly, attempting to help explain why their child was born with anomalies is an important but often overlooked part of the psychosocial support. These families need to move beyond their overwhelming feelings and pay full attention to their child's care.

Many health care providers become actively involved in the care of such children, each with a specific role. The role for the clinical geneticist is straightforward: to determine if the child's anomaly is an isolated defect, or represents one finding as part of a genetic syndrome. There are literally thousands of genetic syndromes, most of which are very rare. Even the more common conditions such as Down syndrome and Williams syndrome, with a prevalence of 1 in 700 and 1 in 20,000, respectively, occur at rates that make it unlikely for most to have a vast experience with them, if any at all. Taken as a group, however, genetic conditions are common enough that a busy practitioner will likely have one or more children with a genetic diagnosis, be it sometimes unrecognized. With a seemingly infinite number of potential diagnoses, it is understandable that most health care providers feel intimidated when presented with a child with a congenital anomaly. It is the purpose of this chapter to eliminate the mystery behind the clinical genetics evaluation, reviewing the clinical geneticist's role, and illustrating how a clinical genetics evaluation can provide valuable information for the parents and other family members as well as the health care team.

THE GENETICS EVALUATION

The genetics evaluation is very similar in format to the standard medical evaluation, as it includes a history and physical exam, and is supplemented by laboratory testing. The genetics evaluation is, however, very different in its execution and emphasis. It is the goal of the next chapters to describe in detail the genetics evaluation of the child with a congenital anomaly, emphasizing how the genetics history, physical examination, and laboratory testing differ from those done in other areas of medical practice. As will be discussed in more detail, it is the subtle findings, be they in the family history or physical exam, that are essential in making the diagnosis of a genetic syndrome.

This chapter reviews how a geneticist evaluates a child with a congenital anomaly and, more importantly, why. Finally, the unique features of the genetics evaluation, especially the genetics physical exam, are covered. Chapter 5 focuses on the classification of various types of birth defects, including how they can be related in a syndrome, a sequence, or an association. Chapter 6 concludes this section by reviewing the array of genetic tests that are currently available to aid in diagnosis, and some that will be available soon. We discuss the strengths of each test, as well as its limitations. The notion of genetic testing often raises concerns for patients and their families that go beyond the medical results, such as issues with cost, insurance discrimination, and even the ethical implications of this testing. These will be addressed in Chapter 7. Finally, Chapter 8 reviews the genetic counseling process, the specialized manner in which genetics professionals interact and communicate with patients and their families.

Indications for a Genetics Referral

One of the more common questions I am asked as a clinical geneticist, by physicians and by parents, is who should be referred for a genetics evaluation. This is a difficult question to answer for several reasons. The physician (or parent) may have a perspective on the case that is not the same as that of a clinical geneticist. For example, subtle findings may not be recognized. A pediatrician may believe that his or her patient has an isolated cleft palate, but the child, in fact, also has additional minor facial differences, which may indicate a genetic syndrome. Or an especially important item in family history may not be recognized by the nongeneticist (e.g., a deaf child's uncle with early-onset gray hair suggests the diagnosis of Waardenberg syndrome), but asking about early-onset gray hair in family members is not something most audiologists are likely to consider in their initial evaluation of a deaf child. Many would ask about visual problems, as they are a common associated finding in some forms of syndromic hearing impairment. However, although it is expected that one would focus on the more severe problems, such as retinitis pigmentosa (which would indicate Usher syndrome), more common ocular conditions may be as important to making a genetic diagnosis. For example, myopia (near sightedness) is very common in the general population, but when it co-occurs with a hearing problem, it may indicate Stickler syndrome or another Type II collagenopathy (see Chapter 9). As is the case with these examples, in most instances, the likelihood of a genetic disorder is greater than the nongenetics professional realizes. Therefore, the "safe" rule for health care professionals is that patients should be referred for a clinical genetics evaluation once the clinical genetics evaluation has been considered. That said, there are several clear indications that should prompt a clinical genetics evaluation. Discussed below, these by no means represent a complete list, but are examples of the more common and obvious indications.

The Child with Multiple Anomalies

It should be obvious that a patient with multiple anomalies is likely to have a genetic syndrome as the underlying and unifying cause for their clinical problems. Few health care professionals would not send such a child for a clinical genetics evaluation. However, it is worth noting that this is not true for the adult patient with multiple congenital anomalies. Often such adults were never evaluated by a clinical geneticist, as such services were not available when they were younger. Or, they may have been evaluated, but no diagnosis was made. In that case a re-evaluation is certainly worthwhile. Each year new genetics syndromes are identified based on novel clinical findings or due to advanced genetic testing techniques. For example, a child with failure to thrive (poor growth) and developmental delay may only develop the physical findings of Williams syndrome later in life (see Williams syndrome). These are discussed in more detail in Chapter 6. Even the oldest genetic test, cytogenetic analysis, has improved in quality substantially in the past decade. For these reasons any patient with multiple anomalies who does not have a diagnosis should be re-evaluated periodically, every 3 to 5 years. This is a general "rule," and applies to any patient that a clinical geneticist sees. In some cases, however, the interval should be even shorter, as we discuss below.

Williams Syndrome

It is important for anyone who cares for children with communication disorders to have some familiarity with Williams syndrome. This is because people with Williams syndrome have a unique deficit in communication skills. Williams syndrome is characterized by supravalvular aortic stenosis, neonatal hypercalcemia, a distinct facial appearance, and a very specific and unique cognitive deficit. Additional findings include short stature, hypothyroidism, strabismus, and a hoarse voice. As individuals age, they are at risk for progressive narrowing of other major arteries, progressive joint stiffness, and bowel and bladder diverticulae.

The physical appearance of people with Williams syndrome changes with age as well. Although the diagnosis may be missed in young children, especially those without a heart defect, the appearance becomes more prominent later in life as the developmental issues become more obvious as well (Figure 4-1).

While most are diagnosed as infants because of the presence of the heart anomaly and/or hypercalcemia, many children with Williams syndrome come to medical attention later in life due to developmental delay. However, the developmental delay seen in Williams syndrome is unique. Expressive language remains intact at a near normal level, but receptive language skills are quite low. This has been termed the "Williams syndrome cognitive profile."

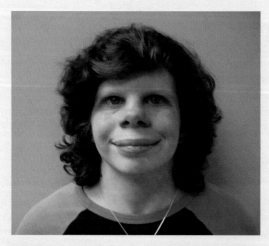

FIGURE 4–1. A 14–year-old girl with Williams syndrome. Note the upturned nasal tip, full low- set cheeks, and wide mouth with full lips.

In addition, Williams syndrome individuals tend to be very friendly, leading to the term "cocktail party personality" to describe the verbal skills and excessive and inappropriate friendliness. Another area of relative strength is long-term memory, and many affected children have an affinity and proficiency for music. Overall, the cognitive level of someone with Williams syndrome typically falls in the moderate mental retardation range, but because of the relatively strong expressive verbal skills, their cognitive ability tends to be overestimated by health care providers and teachers.

Williams syndrome is caused by a microdeletion on chromosome 7q21. The deletion is not visible by standard cytogenetics, requiring a specialized FISH test to identify. Therefore, there must be a clinical suspicion to order the correct test. Among the many genes deleted in this segment is elastin. Elastin deficiency is thought to account for the narrowing of the arteries and joint stiffness. Other genes in the deleted segment are thought to be involved in the cognitive deficits. One such candidate is LIMK1.

For more information, see http://www.geneclinics.org, or http://www.WSPA.org.

The Significance of Minor Anomalies

Another common indication is the patient with a major anomaly who has in addition several minor anomalies. Often, these are facial, and result in the patient having an unusual facial appearance. Such patients are referred to as "dysmorphic," reflecting the fact that their facial appearance is not "normal." Years ago such patients were often referred to as "FLKs," or "funny looking kids." Such terms are strongly discouraged today, but sadly are still used by some professionals who have limited experience with special needs patients, or are themselves insensitive. Such determinations are not based entirely on an individual observer's subjective assessment; those that can be measured, such as eye spacing and ear length, are compared to accepted normal values. (Normal values for anthropomorphic measurements are readily available in the *Handbook of Normal Physical Measurements*.) However, other abnormalities, such as lip contour and ear shape, are based on the viewer's experience, and are therefore somewhat subjective. These subtle abnormal findings are referred to as "minor anomalies," distinguishing them from more severe congenital anomalies, which are termed "major anomalies" (see Major and Minor Anomalies). Examples of minor anomalies are provided in Figure 4-2. As is discussed in the following section, these subtle findings often are the most valuable to the clinical geneticist in making a diagnosis.

Major and Minor Anomalies

Structural birth defects and congenital anomalies can be classified several different ways. One is based on the underlying pathogenesis (reviewed in detail in Chapter 5), while another is based on severity. When differentiated by severity, congenital anomalies fall into two main categories: major and minor. A *major anomaly* is one that has significant medical or cosmetic consequences, such as a congenital heart defect, cleft lip, or craniosynostosis. In contrast, a *minor anomaly* represents a clinically insignificant departure from normal development. Although it may indicate an underlying syndrome (see text), a minor anomaly has no direct adverse affect on the person's medical well-being. Examples of minor anomalies include widely set eyes, single palmar creases, and birth marks. Minor external anomalies are most commonly found in areas where features are complex and variable, such as the face, external ears, hands, and feet.

It is important to recognize that minor and major anomalies are not limited to physical defects, but also include neurodevelopmental abnormalities, such as mental retardation and psychiatric disease, and disorders of physical development, such as short stature.

An Isolated Anomaly

As discussed above, a clinical genetics evaluation is considered by most health care providers to be a valuable effort for a patient with multiple anomalies. This is due to its relatively high rate of success in identifying an underlying genetic syndrome. However, the utility of such an evaluation in a patient with an isolated anomaly is not as clear. Most isolated anomalies are multifactorial in that they are caused by genetic and nongenetic factors (see Chapter 3). For most, such as orofacial clefting (see Chapter 10), the genetic factors are at best incompletely understood, and clinically useful genetic testing is not available. However, most isolated conditions are heterogeneous, and a subset of cases are entirely caused by genetic factors, and demonstrate a Mendelian inheritance pattern. For a rapidly growing number, genetic research has made great progress in identifying the genetic basis. In such cases, clinical genetic testing is often available and important in the evaluation of these patients. Hearing impairment is one such example, and is discussed in more detail throughout the book, but especially in Chapter 9. For isolated anomalies, a genetics evaluation serves several important functions. First, it confirms the isolated nature of the anomaly, as subtle findings are sought that may be over-

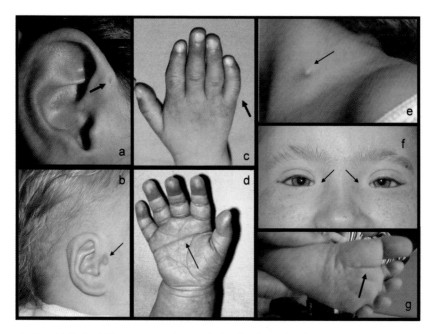

FIGURE 4–2. Minor anomalies: **A.** Helical pit. **B.** Pre-auricular ear tag. **C.** 5th finger clinodactyly. **D.** Single palmar crease. **E.** Neck tag. **F.** Epicanthal folds. **G.** Deep vertical plantar increase. Each of these may be associated with a genetic syndrome, or be present in an otherwise normal individual. (Images A–F, Courtesy of Raoul CM Hennekam, ICH, London.)

looked by nongenetics professionals. Second, the genetics professional (medical geneticist or genetic counselor) can discuss genetic testing options, arrange for the testing to be done, and counsel on the test results. This process is discussed in more detail in Chapters 7 and 8. One key aspect to recognize is that one must make every effort to stay current with the state of biomedical research for each area, as disease-associated genes are being uncovered at a rapid rate.

Finally, even for isolated anomalies for which no genetic testing exists, a genetic evaluation can offer at least a review of the empiric recurrence risk data. This is also discussed in Chapter 9, Genetics and Hearing Loss.

The Patient with Developmental Delay

One of the most common reasons for a geneticist to see a patient, particularly a child, is developmental delays. There are many book chapters and review articles that provide a more complete discussion of this topic, and some are listed at the end of this chapter. Suffice it to say here that every child with a developmental delay of unknown etiology should be seen by a geneticist at least once. Numerous genetic syndromes have developmental delay as one finding, and for many the other associated findings can be very subtle. Among the most common is Fragile X syndrome, with an incidence estimated as high as 1 in 2000 males. Although Fragile X syndrome has a classic phenotypic presentation (Figure 4–3), a substantial percentage of affected patients have few if any associated findings. Among the more common but subtle associated findings are large ears, an elongated facial appearance, large testicles, and a family history of females with premature ovarian failure (entering menopause before age 40 years of age). For that reason, Fragile X testing is routine for all children with developmental delay.

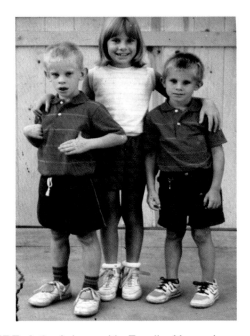

FIGURE 4–3. A boy with Fragile X syndrome (*left*), with his older sister and fraternal twin brother. Note the relatively tall stature, with a large head and long face, protruding ears, and prominent jaw. Fragile X syndrome is among the most common causes of mental retardation in males, occurring in 1 per 2000-6000. It has a complex genetic inheritance and underlying genetic mechanism due to an expansion of a repeated DNA sequence on the X chromosome. For more information, see http://www.Geneclinics.org, or http://www.fragilex.org. (Reprinted with permission from *Archives of Pediatric and Adolescent Medicine, 152,* p. 89. Copyright © 1998. American Medical Association. All rights reserved.)

Loss of Developmental Milestones

A child who presents with a loss of developmental milestones suggests a specific category of disorders, those that are progressive and actively worsen. For reasons that will be discussed below, it is common for a child with developmental delay to be labeled as having a "loss of milestones." This mistake can be very detrimental when trying to make a diagnosis, as that label suggests a much different and narrower set of diagnostic possibilities than typical developmental delay. "Loss of developmental milestones" suggests an exact scenario—a child who can no longer do a skill that he or she had previously mastered: he or she could walk, or speak in sentences, but now cannot. Identifying a loss of developmental milestones suggests a particular category of diseases such as lysosomal storage disease or Rett syndrome.

Most developmental delay is secondary to a static process. The underlying neurologic impairment is *not* progressive, and does not change. It may, however, not be recognized as such. As a child ages, he or she is expected to make progress and acquire new skills. The impairment may manifest only as the child ages, and the new skills that are expected to be obtained are not. For example, the child may have sat at an age that falls within the expected range, but stands later than normal, and walks at an even later time. To the parent, it will seem as if their child was developmentally normal for those first few months, and then became abnormal. Furthermore, the degree of delay will only increase with time, as additional milestones are not met. Therefore, parents will erroneously believe that the child's problems are progressive in nature, and may present it as such to their pediatrician. If this mistaken notion is not recognized, it will lead the health care team to consider an incorrect group of conditions.

Family History

As discussed above, a detailed family history often reveals information that suggests the presence of a genetic disorder. This is especially true when there is a family history of the same condition seen in the patient, even when that condition is not commonly thought of as a "genetic disorder." One common example is an isolated cleft lip and palate. As discussed earlier, and in more detail in Chapter 10, isolated cleft lip and palate is a multifactorial trait. However, a subset has a strong genetic determination, and follows a Mendelian inheritance pattern, often autosomal dominant with incomplete penetrance.

It is important to remember that not all conditions that occur in multiple family members are genetic. Some are due to nongenetic factors that also cluster in families, such as shared environments. Conditions that occur in families but are not caused by genetic factors are labeled "pseudogenetic." The classic example is a family with multiple children with mental retardation and dysmorphic facial appearance due to repeated maternal alcohol use during the pregnancies. Each child has Fetal Alcohol syndrome. Although most physicians and scientists agree that alcohol abuse has clear genetic underpinnings, the children in this example have a common phenotype due to their shared environmental influence.

The Benefits of Making a Genetic Diagnosis

As discussed above, a genetics evaluation can be quite complex, involving detailed medical and family histories, a specialized physical examination, and genetic testing. The goal, however, is simple: to determine if the patient's anomaly is isolated, or represents one component finding of an underlying genetic syndrome. One common and unfortunate misconception is that such a determination is pointless. This sentiment is reflected in comments such as "What good will it do to have that label?" "You can't fix it" "What difference does it make?"

There is some truth to these comments. Most anomalies cannot be undone using genetic therapies, nor does having a genetic diagnosis significantly alter how many are treated. However, for an increasing number of genetically determined anomalies, accurate identification of the genetic cause may alter management. It will certainly change the patient's overall care. Furthermore, making a correct genetic diagnosis will permit accurate prognostic and recurrence risk counseling, more informed management decisions, and the identification of appropriate social support resources. These are discussed in detail in in Chapter 1. To illustrate the significance of making a genetic diagnosis, let us consider an infant boy with a cleft palate (CP). If that child's CP is isolated (e.g., not associated with any other birth defects or underlying genetic syndrome), the child has an excellent prognosis. He will need one or more surgeries on his palate, long-term speech therapy, and eventually orthodontic treatments. However, he is not at increased risk for unrelated medical problems and should have normal intelligence and a favorable long-term outcome. Assuming that there is no family history of similar or related problems, his parents would have a low likelihood of having another child with a cleft, approximately 1 to 3% with each subsequent pregnancy. His risk for an offspring with CP is similarly low.

However, this all changes if the CP was due to an underlying genetic syndrome, such as Del22q11.2, or velocardiofacial syndrome (VCFS; see Chapter 10). In this case, the child will be at risk for significant learning, behavioral, and psychiatric problems, as well as a long list of medical complications, such as congenital heart disease, immune deficiency, and endocrine dysfunction. The likelihood that his parents would have another affected child would range from 50% if one parent is also affected with Del22q11.2, to under 1%, if both were normal. His risk is 50% for each child he fathers.

Children with VCFS are at risk for vascular anomalies, including aberrant placement of the carotid arteries so that they course near the potential surgical field for a cleft palate repair. This is obviously something a plastic surgeon would want to know prior to surgery.

Furthermore, children with VCFS have a poor response rate to speech therapy, and often manifest velopharyngeal insufficiency even after aggressive therapy post cleft palate repair.

HOW TO IDENTIFY A GENETIC SYNDROME/ MAKE A DIAGNOSIS

Now that it has been established that there is a clear benefit to making a genetic diagnosis, we review *how* to make a diagnosis. How does a clinical geneticist sort through the information obtained through the medical and family histories and physical exam to reach a genetic syndrome diagnosis?

The traditional approach to identifying an underlying genetic syndrome in the field of medical genetics begins with careful personal and family medical histories, including prenatal and birth histories, followed by a detailed physical exam. A detailed medical history is essential, as it is vital to know each medical issue, even (especially!) those that may seem unrelated to what is viewed as the primary problem. For example, a history of myopia in a child with cleft palate may not seem to be connected, but it suggests a diagnosis of Stickler syndrome. Similarly, a family history must also include identifying all of the information relevant to the primary problem. For example, for a child with a cleft palate, questions about absence of dentition or speech problems in other family members are important. However, it is also important to be thorough and ask about any other medical problems in family members. First, such questions may reveal information that would point to a correct diagnosis. One such example would be myopia and early-onset arthritis in family members of the child with the cleft palate, which suggest the diagnosis of Stickler syndrome. A second reason is that another genetic problem may be identified that is truly unrelated to the primary indication for evaluation. For example, it is not that uncommon to identify a strong family history of early onset breast and ovarian cancer that suggests a BRCA1- or BRCA2-related cancer susceptibility syndrome. In such cases, a referral to a cancer genetics clinic should be recommended, with the clear acknowledgment that this is separate from the other anomaly.

The Genetics Physical Examination

The genetics physical exam is different in many ways from the usual physical exam. The emphasis of this exam is not on the health of the patient, but is focused on subtle physical findings that represent clues to the underlying genetic syndrome. This approach is termed "dysmorphology," which is the study of abnormal form with an emphasis on structural developmental abnormalities. A dysmorphologic evaluation of a child (or fetus or adult) looks for unusual physical (or behavioral) characteristics that might provide insight into errors in embryologic or fetal development. Anomalies that may lead to the suspicion of a particular unifying diagnosis may be *major* or *minor* (see p. 48). It is important to remember that minor anomalies are important only in the context within which they are viewed. For example, single palmar creases occur in up to 4% of the general population. If seen in an otherwise healthy individual, they have little importance. However, when seen in a hypotonic newborn with a flattened midface, upslanting eyes, and an atrial-ventricular canal, the diagnosis of Down syndrome should be strongly considered.

Significance of Minor Anomalies

The best clues are the rarest. . . . Quite often, these are not the most obvious anomalies nor even the ones that have the greatest significance for the patient's health.

John Aase, M.D.

Minor anomalies, by definition, have little to no medical significance. However, as stated in Dr. Aase's quote above, it is through the identification of minor anomalies that most genetic syndrome diagnoses are made. However, it is also essential to remember that minor anomalies are only significant in the context in which they are seen—a patient suspected of having a genetic syndrome. Studies have shown about 14% of babies have a single minor anomaly. However, with more minor anomalies, the likelihood of an associated major anomaly rises. The 0.8% of infants with two minor anomalies had a fivefold higher rate of having a major defect than the general group, with likelihood of having a major anomaly rising from 20 to 90% for the 0.5% of infants with three or more minor anomalies (Leppig, Werler, Cann, Cook, & Holmes, 1987; Marden, Smith, & McDonald, 1964; Mehes, Mestyan, Knoch, & Vinceller, 1973). Although a single minor anomaly may have no significance, the presence of three or more should prompt a search for a major anomaly, and an evaluation for a genetic syndrome.

Now that the significance of minor anomalies is evident, the next question is: How can one distinguish a normal variant from a minor anomaly? In fact, that is one of the most difficult chores for the clinical geneticist, and debates persist for various structures. This is a question that clinical geneticists still debate. A complete catalogue is being developed by Dr. Raoul H. Hennekam, Professor of Clinical Genetics and Dysmorphology at Great Ormond Street Hospital for Children in London, England. Finally, it is important to realize that many genetic syndromes have characteristic findings that are not physical (see How to Make the Diagnosis of a Genetic Syndrome and Figure 3-13).

How to Make the Diagnosis of a Genetic Syndrome

JC is a 3-month-old boy with feeding difficulty due to a large tongue. He had a small omphamocele repaired (a birth defect in which the intestines protrude through the umbilicus) that was easily corrected by surgery on day 3 of life. His mother's pregnancy history was uncomplicated until she entered early labor at 34 weeks. JC had trouble breathing after birth due to the large tongue, but that has resolved somewhat. Now, the primary issue is that the large tongue interferes with feeding. The only other noteworthy finding is that JC was very large at birth, weighing 3530 grams (above the 95% for 34 weeks gestation). On physical exam JC remains large, despite the poor feeding. His tongue is large for his mouth, but he is otherwise normal in appearance except for deep creases that cross his ear lobes.

How to Proceed to Make a Genetic Diagnosis?

There are, of course, many different accepted methods that are used to diagnose a genetic syndrome in a child with multiple anomalies. My personal method is to first identify the most unusual anomaly and develop a differential diagnosis of possible syndromes from that. In this case, the omphalocele is the finding to key on. From that point on, one can use either textbooks (e.g., *Smith's Recognizable Pattern of Human Malformation*) or computer databases (London Dysmorphology Database), to find what syndromes are associated with omphalocele. This would generate a list of a dozen or so syndromes. Next, see what syndromes from that list are associated with large size, and/or a large tongue. This narrows the list to a small number, with the most likely being Beckwith-Wiedemann syndrome. This is further supported by the fact that earlobe creases are common in Beckwith-Wiedemann syndrome, but not in any other syndrome on that list.

 The diagnosis is significant, as children with Beckwith-Wiedemann syndrome are at increased risk for developing a variety of tumors. Otherwise, most children with Beckwith-Wiedemann syndrome are healthy, and taller than their peers. Intelligence is normal. Genetic testing is available, but will only pick up about 60% of cases, so a negative test does not rule out the disorder.

 To review, this method involves: (1) careful observation of the major (omphalocele, large tongue) and minor (earlobe creases) anomalies; (2) identification of the most unusual of the findings;

(3) use of a textbook or database to develop a list of possible syndromes; (4) adding in additional findings to continually whittle down the list to a manageable few syndromes; (5) thoroughly reviewing the limited number of syndromes to determine which one is the best fit; and (6) if it exists, ordering testing (genetic or other) to confirm the diagnosis.

This is a relatively straightforward method to make a genetic syndrome diagnosis. Of course, it is not always so simple (if it were, clinical geneticists would all be out of work), but it provides a framework to at least begin the process.

REFERENCES

Leppig, K. A., Werler, M. M., Cann, C. I., Cook, C. A., & Holmes, L. B. (1987). Predictive value of minor anomalies. Association with major malformations. *Journal of Pediatrics, 110*, 531-537.

Marden. P. M., Smith, D. W., & McDonald, M. J. (1964) Congenital anomalies in the newborn infant, including minor variations. A study of 4,412 babies by surface examination for anomalies and buccal smear for sex chromatin. *Journal of Pediatrics, 64*, 357-371.

Mehes, K., Mestyan, J., Knoch, V., & Vinceller, M. (1973). Minor malformation in the neonate. *Helv Pediatr Acta, 28*, 477-483.

RECOMMENDED READING

Aase, J. M. (1990). *Diagnostic dysmorphology.* New York: Plenum.

Cohen, M. M. (1997). *The child with multiple birth defects* (2nd ed.). New York: Oxford University Press.

Robin, N. H. (2006). It does matter. The importance of making the diagnosis of a genetic syndrome. *Current Opinion in Pediatrics, 18*(6), 595-597.

For more information on Rett syndrome, see http://www.rettsyndrome.org

For more information on lysosomal storage diseases, see http://www.lysosomallearn ing.com

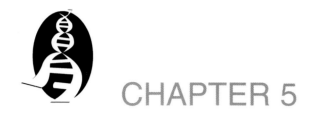

CHAPTER 5

Classification of Birth Defects

MARNI J. FALK, MD
NATHANIEL H. ROBIN, MD

INTRODUCTION

The previous chapter reviewed the medical geneticists' approach to the patient with a congenital anomaly, emphasizing the need for careful data collection through detailed history taking and the specialized "dysmorphologic" physical exam. This chapter reviews how these structural anomalies are categorized based on the pathogenic mechanism. This is a crucial step in the assessment of these patients, as this determination will affect prognosis, treatment, management, and recurrence risk estimates. Furthermore, this approach includes understanding how various findings, including both major and minor anomalies, are related to each another. This may then lead to identification of a specific genetic etiology or category of disease. Increasingly, genetic testing is available for confirmation of these clinical diagnoses. This topic is covered in the following chapter.

BIRTH DEFECTS

Birth defects are common. They occur in every population, even in the absence of known risk factors such as family history, ethnicity, or parental age. Overall, about 1% to 3% of *all newborns* have a significant congenital anomaly that will interfere with normal functioning if left uncorrected. Furthermore, congenital defects are a leading cause of neonatal morbidity in developed countries, outpacing prematurity and infection, and they represent a significant contributor to neonatal morbidity and mortality.

Chapter 4 reviewed the systematic approach toward identifying the etiology of a congenital anomaly, but one important issue is to determine if the anomaly or anomalies present are isolated to a single region of the body, such as the craniofacial region, or involve other regions or organ systems. Approximately two thirds of all anomalies are limited to a single system, whereas smaller percentages are part of a multiple malformation syndrome, sequence, association, or complex. A particularly useful classification scheme for birth defects that provides a general framework for discussion about the etiology, and therefore prognostic information, is based on pathogenic mechanism. There are four main mechanistic categories of birth defects: deformation, disruption, malformation, and dysplasia (Figure 5-1).

Deformation

A *deformation* refers to an abnormal structure in which the developmental program was normal, but the structure is now abnormal in appearance due to abnormal mechanical forces that have distorted the structure. These problems often arise late in gestation once the structure has already formed (e.g., after the first trimester), but still may have severe effects on a structure's configuration and function. Most deformational anomalies involve cartilage, bone, and joints as these tissues are more likely to yield to intrauterine pressure. Such pressure can be extrinsic to the fetus, or intrinsic. Extrinsic factors are those in which the abnormal forces that cause the anomaly arise outside the fetus. Several types of extrinsic factors can cause intrauterine fetal constraint. Some are purely maternal and space-related, including a primigravida, a structural uterine abnormality (fibroids, bicornuate uterus), and multiple gestations producing crowding. Others arise from an underlying medical problem. Oligohydramnios (low amniotic fluid levels), due to either maternal/placental problems or decreased fetal urine output (for any one of the many possible reasons, including absent fetal kidneys or a blocked urinary tract) is one example. Oligohydramnios results in a complex referred to as "Potter's sequence" in which a fetus/infant manifests flat facies, low-set ears, a recessed jaw, lung hypoplasia, and joint contractures (Figure 5-2). Finally, some deformations are caused by "internal" forces. One example would be a case of clubbed feet associated with holoprosencephaly (a brain malformation). The genetic and

A. **NORMAL DEVELOPMENT**

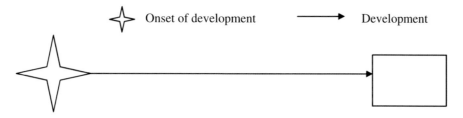

B. **MALFORMATION** = Early developmental error prevents normal structure formation

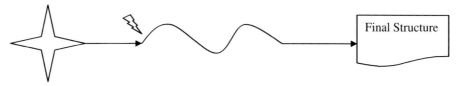

C. **DEFORMATION** = Mechanical force alters normally-formed structure

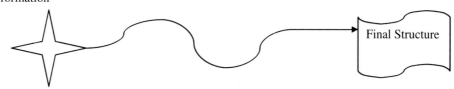

D. **DISRUPTION** = Abrupt interruption of normal development by a physiologic or mechanical force

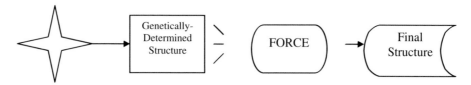

E. **DYSPLASIA** = Tissue-specific abnormality

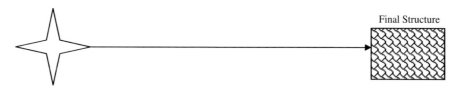

FIGURE 5–1. Categories of congenital anomaly pathogenesis.

developmental programs for the feet were normal, and the feet were normally formed. However, the aberrant neurological signals sent by the dysmorphic brain to the muscles surrounding the feet led to the feet becoming contorted.

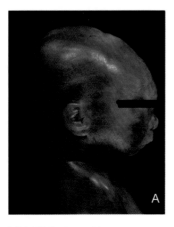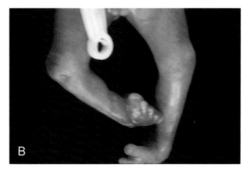

FIGURE 5–2. Potters sequence. **A.** Note the flat nasal bridge, low-set and posteriorly rotated ears, and recessed chin; **B.** Note the lower limb contractures due to oligohydramnios. (Photo courtesy of Dr. Ona Faye-Petersen.)

Deformations potentially have a favorable prognosis. In contrast to malformations, which are fixed once they occur, deformations often will begin to correct spontaneously once the abnormal mechanical stress is removed. For some deformations, such as fetal crowding, the abnormal stress is removed with birth. For others, such as the abnormal neurologic tone, the force cannot be removed, and the prognosis is less favorable. Treatments such as bracing or physical therapy often are required to produce an opposite corrective stress to that of the force. Over months to years, differential growth often occurs in the affected body part that may allow the deformation to gradually disappear.

Deformations often are isolated, without association with mental impairment or other medical problems. In such cases, the recurrence risk is low unless structural anomalies are identified within the mother's uterus. However, they can also co-occur with other anomalies in the context of a genetic syndrome. One such example is the deformations seen in Potters sequence, which is secondary to underdeveloped kidneys, all part of branchio-oto-renal syndrome.

Disruption

The second type of birth defect is a *disruption.* Similar to a deformation, a disruption involves a structure for which the genetic program was intact and development proceeded normally. However, during development, or after it is formed, the structure is damaged. The most common mechanism is a vascular insult, in which the blood supply to the structure is interrupted. This can occur due to an external event, such as in amniotic band sequence (see Amniotic Band Sequence and Disruptions), or internal, such as a vasospasm caused by fetal cocaine exposure.

Amniotic Band Sequence and Disruptions

Amniotic band sequence (ABS) is the term applied to congenital anomalies that occur in association with fibrous bands. These bands typically arise from the placenta, and are thought to "strangle" the affected structure, causing the blood supply to be interrupted, and the structure to be destroyed. Anomalies seen in ABS are therefore **disruptions**. They are typically asymmetric limb reductions, but the severity can be merely a cosmetic to a lethal cranial defect (Figure 5–3A and 5–3B). Although these anomalies can be similar to what is seen with a **malformation**, certain characteristics suggest the ABS mechanism. These include asymmetric involvement of the limbs, the transverse nature of the reduction defects, and the presence of an otherwise normally formed fetus or child. The finding of additional associated anomalies, such as cleft palate, or a congenital heart defect, likely suggests another diagnosis (Robin, Franklin, Prucka, Ryan, & Grant, 2005).

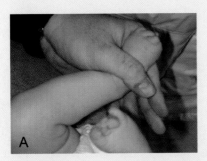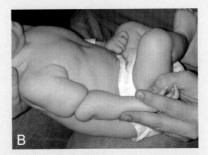

FIGURE 5–3. Amniotic band sequence. **A.** amputation of several toes and **B.** a constriction ring around the upper arm. (Reprinted with permission of Wiley-Liss, Inc. a subsidiary of John Wiley & Sons, Inc. from "Clefting, Amniotic Bands, and Polydactyly: A Distinct Phenotype That Supports an Intrinsic Mechanism for Amniotic Band Sequence," by N. H. Robin, J. Franklin, S. Prucka, A. B. Ryan, and J. H. Grant, 2005. *American Journal of Medical Genetics, 137A,* 298–301.)

Both disruptions and malformations cause abnormal structures, and it is often difficult to discern which mechanism caused the anomaly. Disruptions can be differentiated from malformations by the fact that a disruption will affect multiple different tissue types within a well-defined anatomic region which do not necessarily fit expected developmental boundaries. For example, amniotic bands slice through all layers of a fetus' skin, soft tissue, muscle, and bone regardless of their embryologic relationship. Similarly, physiological disruptions such as ischemia or hemorrhage damage all tissues in the region. As is the case with deformations, disruptions are seldom associated with intrinsic tissue defects, mental impairment, or other separate medical problems, such as a congenital heart defect. Their recurrence risk typically is low unless an underlying genetic etiology is detected as cause for the inciting event. One such example is genetically determined clotting disorders, called thrombophilias, which can cause repeated in utero clotting. Similarly, repeat maternal cocaine use results in multiple pregnancies at risk for disruptions.

Malformation

Malformations are the most common category of congenital anomaly, and are what most people think of when they think of a birth defect. A malformation results from failure or inadequate completion of one or more early embryonic developmental processes, such as cellular proliferation, differentiation, induction, apoptosis, fusion between adjacent tissues, or the correct sequence of developmental events. Identifying an anomaly as a malformation implies that the error occurred early in development when tissues were differentiating or organ systems were forming, as it is unlikely for a true malformation to occur in the later fetal period when most organ systems are already formed. A malformation can result from intrinsic errors in the developmental program itself, as caused by chromosomal alterations, gene mutations, or epigenetic alterations such as DNA methylation abnormalities. Teratogens interfering with an otherwise normal genetic program at a critical time in development can also result in a malformation. However, the most common etiology for a malformation is multifactorial, an interaction with one or more genetic and nongenetic (environmental) factors. This is discussed in more detail in Chapter 3. Orofacial clefting, including cleft lip and cleft palate, is one of the best known examples of a multifactorial trait.

Like most cases of clefting, malformations may occur as a single anomaly. However, several malformations may be present in one person. They may be limited to a particular anatomic region and have effects on a single organ system, such as is the case with Treacher Collins syndrome, in which the findings are limited to the craniofacial skeleton (see Chapter 11, Figure 11–15). Many other syndromes manifest malformations in multiple different organ systems. Velocardiofacial syndrome is one such example (see Chapter 10).

Dysplasia

Dysplasia is the final pathogenic category relevant to the formation of congenital anomalies. This involves intrinsically abnormal cellular organization or function within a specific tissue type that occurs throughout the body.

This may or may not result in a visible structural change. For example, although the bones of a person with achondroplasia are clearly abnormal, those of someone with osteogenesis imperfecta may have a normal external appearance. As opposed to the three other categories of pathogenesis, a dysplasia can produce clinical effects that may persist or worsen throughout life as long as the affected tissue continues to grow or function. This is because dysplasias often involve the genes for proteins that make up the extracellular matrix, or are involved in its maintenance. The extracellular matrix is the "scaffolding" on which the body's structures are made. The components are constantly being made, broken down, and remade over the person's life, so the effect of an abnormal gene and its protein product will be manifest over time. Examples of dysplasias include skeletal osteogenesis imperfecta in which there is abnormal type I collagen, as well as ectodermal dysplasias affecting skin, tooth, hair, and nail development such as Rapp-Hodgkin syndrome (Figure 5-4).

CLINICAL PATTERNS OF CONGENITAL ANOMALIES

The clinical implications of congenital abnormalities vary considerably depending on the context in which they occur. Most birth defects are malformations that involve a localized segment of an organ system or structure. For example, a cleft palate involves the soft palate, which is one part of the craniofacial region. These defects are often identical whether they occur as an isolated anomaly or as part of a syndrome. However, isolated defects do not usually

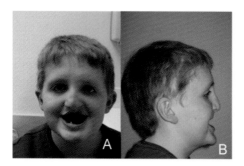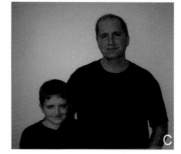

FIGURE 5–4. Rapp-Hodgkin syndrome. **A.** and **B.** Note the repaired cleft, conical teeth, and coarse scalp hair and eyebrows. **C.** With his more mildly affected father, who manifests sparse and coarse scalp hair. (Reprinted with permission of Wiley-Liss, Inc. a subsidiary of John Wiley & Sons, Inc. from "Clefting, Amniotic Bands, and Polydactyly: A Distinct Phenotype That Supports an Intrinsic Mechanism for Amniotic Band Sequence," by N. H. Robin, J. Franklin, S. Prucka, A. B. Ryan, and J. H. Grant, 2005. *American Journal of Medical Genetics, 137A*, 298–301.

follow classic Mendelian inheritance patterns that would be expected if they were caused by a single mutant gene. Rather, they occur more randomly among family members and are thought to result from a multifactorial etiology (see Chapter 3). However, when multiple congenital anomalies are seen in one patient, they can be divided into a category based on the relative frequency with which the component features are seen together and whether a known etiology exists to explain all or some of the features. The categories are syndromes, associations, sequences, and complexes.

Syndrome

A *syndrome* is a set of multiple anomalies that occur in a consistent and recognizable pattern and result from a common pathogenic etiology, which may or may not be genetic. It is important to remember that identifying a syndrome often provides only a useful descriptive label, and does not necessarily identify the underlying etiology. For example, Down syndrome was described in 1920 by Langdon Down. He recognized a similar clinical phenotype of mental retardation, hypotonia, cardiac defects, and a characteristic facial appearance. Only with the later discovery that the cause of this constellation of findings in all affected individuals was the presence of a third copy of chromosome 21 was it proven that a common etiology accounts for the wide variety of seemingly unrelated anomalies seen in individuals with Down syndrome. Although the eponym "Down syndrome" has survived, it is generally preferred that once the underlying cause is identified, such a name should be replaced with a name more representative of the underlying problem, such as Trisomy 21 syndrome in this example. Another example is Rapp-Hodgkin syndrome (see Figure 5–4). This autosomal dominant syndrome is characterized by mixed clefting, ectodermal dysplasia (absent sweat glands, sparse coarse hair, and dystrophic nails).

Thousands of genetic syndromes have been identified. Learning the component features of each syndrome by rote memorization is impractical and daunting. Furthermore, no one clinical feature is pathognomonic for a specific syndrome. A catalogued overview of genetic syndromes is available in multiple texts and Web sites listed in Chapter 4, with individual case reports and specific syndrome reviews available in medical genetics journals such as the *American Journal of Medical Genetics, American Journal of Human Genetics, Journal of Medical Genetics,* and *European Journal of Genetics,* to name a few. A practical approach to fitting seemingly unrelated congenital anomalies into a unifying syndromic diagnosis is to use a reference book that categorizes its glossary by individual anomalies and lists specific syndromes having each feature. By cross-referencing which syndromes appear repeatedly under multiple features present in a particular patient, one can begin to narrow the differential diagnosis. Computer programs such as the Oxford Medical Database help to efficiently achieve similar results.

Association

Like a malformation, an *association* is the term used to reflect a constellation of anomalies that occur together more often than predicted by random chance alone. However, unlike a syndrome, the anomalies seen in an association do not have a recognized unifying cause, such as a chromosomal abnormality (e.g., an extra chromosome 21 in a child with Down syndrome) or genetic mutation (e.g., the Pro250Arg mutation in FGFR3 seen in Muenke type cranio-synostosis (see Chapter 11).

The best known example of an association is VACTERL. VACTERL is an acronym for a **v**ertebral anomalies, **a**nal atresia, **c**ardiac malformations, **t**racheo**e**sophageal fistula, **r**enal anomalies, and **l**imb defects. These anomalies occur in a nonrandom manner, meaning that an individual who has a tracheo-esophageal fistula is more likely to have a renal anomaly than would be expected by chance alone. An affected individual would not be expected to have all of the component findings for a specific association, but the presence of one anomaly should prompt further investigation for other hidden abnormalities that may fit the larger pattern.

By definition, the underlying cause of an association is not known. If the underlying cause is identified, the condition then becomes a syndrome. This occurred recently for CHARGE association. CHARGE is another acronym— **c**oloboma of the eye; congenital **h**eart anomaly; choanal **a**tresia; **r**etardation of mental development and physical growth; **g**enito-urinary anomalies; **e**ar abnormalities and/or deafness. It was originally described by Pagon, Graham, Zonana, and Young in 1981 as an association, with no known unifying cause. Recently, a genetic basis for CHARGE was identified, as mutations in the CHD7 gene have been identified in the majority of CHARGE patients (Lalani et al., 2006). With a genetic basis identified, this condition is now called CHARGE syndrome.

In general, the recurrence risk for an association is low, whereas the prognosis depends on the severity of the defects that are present as well as the potential to correct them.

Sequence

A *sequence* is a pattern of congenital anomalies that result secondarily to the occurrence of a single anomaly. On initial inspection, it may seem that the anomalies are unrelated due to the differences of structures affected. In a sequence, the primary malformation exerts an effect that causes an interference or interruption in the normal developmental process, so that by birth a child appears to have multiple distinct abnormalities involving different areas and organ systems. However, the entire pattern of structural and physiologic consequences can be traced back to derive from a single developmental error. Perhaps the best known is Pierre Robin sequence, which is comprised classically of the triad micrognathia or retrognathia, a "U"-shaped cleft palate, and macroglossia, causing glossoptosis (choking on the tongue) (Figure 5–5). It arises during early development from the primary anomaly of a small or recessed jaw, which then causes superior displacement of the tongue, which interferes with proper closure of the soft palate at 9 weeks. Then, after birth, the relatively large tongue causes glossoptosis.

It is important to distinguish sequences from other multiple anomaly patterns because an isolated sequence carries a lower risk for other systemic anomalies and lower recurrence risk. However, it is important to realize that a sequence can be part of a syndrome as well. For example, about half of Pierre Robin sequence cases are part of a larger syndrome, which is found to be Stickler syndrome in about 50%, and another 25% is Del22q11 (velocardiofacial) syndrome (see Chapter 11 for more information on these disorders).

Field Defect (Complex)

A *field defect,* or *complex,* consists of congenital anomalies that appear to have occurred in structures that, at a certain stage of development, were located in close proximity, or were particularly vulnerable at the same time, and were similarly affected by some pathologic event. The underlying cause of most developmental field complexes is unknown. Early literature suggested a vascular disruption as a common cause, such as aberrant blood vessel formation that resulted in absence or hypoplasia of developing structures normally supplied by those vessels. In addition, localized hemorrhage resulting from vascular rupture can damage adjacent tissues through pressure effects, hypoxia or starvation at critical developmental junctures, or biochemical reactions

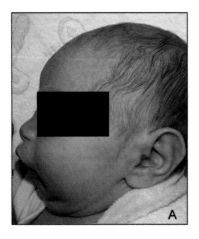
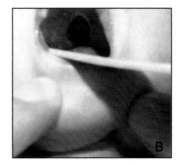

FIGURE 5–5. Pierre Robin sequence. **A.** Note the small jaw with the low-set and posteriorly rotated ear. **B.** The associated "U"-shaped cleft palate. (Courtesy Dr. Robert J. Shprintzen.)

with extravasated blood. This mechanism has been implicated in the pathogenesis of hemifacial microsomia in animal models, but later studies have suggested that the more likely mechanism involves inhibited migration of neural crest cells (see Goldenhar Syndrome).

PHENOCOPIES

When fitting multiple congenital anomalies into a larger clinical pattern it is important to consider potential phenocopies. These entities appear to have an underlying genetic etiology, but in actuality are caused by environmental factors or stochastic variation. For example, valproic acid embryopathy or retinoic acid embryopathy can cause similar patterns of anomalies as might be seen with Trisomy 18 syndrome or DiGeorge syndrome, respectively. Similarly, familial mental retardation can occur in families with multiple generations of alcoholism, or in cases of maternal phenlyketonuria. In this instance, the fetus is only a carrier for the condition; it is the mother who is affected. In addition, disorders that occur with high population frequency with increasing age might appear to follow a Mendelian inheritance pattern when multiple family members are affected, as with coronary artery disease or breast cancer. A genetic etiology should be suspected in complex traits with increasing severity of the disease, when the less frequently affected sex is affected, or when an individual is affected at a younger age than is commonly associated with a specific disorder.

THE ROLE OF GENETIC TESTING

Once the likely pathogenesis of anomalies is determined and the clinical pattern of congenital malformations is identified, the ability to rationally proceed with diagnostic testing becomes clearer. Deformational anomalies seldom require any laboratory-based diagnostic evaluation. Suspected disruptions may prompt investigation for an underlying thrombophilia (increased susceptibility to clot) if an intrauterine vascular event is suspected as in the case of a fetal cerebrovascular accident or limb anomaly. Dysplasias would require a more focused diagnostic evaluation depending on the tissue type affected. For example, if the dysmorphologic evaluation detects coarse facial features and hepatosplenomegaly, further metabolic screening for a storage disorder would be indicated. It is useful to consult with a metabolic specialist to facilitate a comprehensive evaluation potentially requiring costly screening blood tests, invasive tissue biopsies for cytological staining and enzyme analysis, or DNA-based genetic assays when considering dysplasias. These will be discussed in more detail in Chapter 6.

Goldenhar Syndrome (Oculoauriculovertebral Spectrum)

Goldenhar syndrome, oculoauriculovertebral spectrum, and hemifacial microsomia are all names applied to the constellation of findings that includes facial asymmetry due to asymmetric maxillary and mandibular hypoplasia, ipsilateral microtia with associated preauricular skin pits and tags; epibulbar dermoids of the cornea; and a wide range of extracranial malformations, such as vertebral, cardiac, and renal defects (Figure 5–6). Obviously, the clinical spectrum of this condition is very wide, and the different names have been used to describe different presentations. Goldenhar syndrome is often used to describe cases with more severe involvement, whereas hemifacial microsomia typically refers to patients in whom manifestations are limited to craniofacial asymmetry. Oculoauriculovertebral spectrum is the name used by many to refer to the entire spectrum, as this reflects the fact that this is not a discrete syndrome, but a spectrum of findings.

With such a wide range of clinical presentations, it is not surprising that OAV is etiologically heterogeneous, with many genetic and nongenetic causes described. Included in this long list are maternal diabetes (diabetic embryopathy), prenatal exposure to retinoic acid, and chromosomal imbalances, such as trisomy 7 mosaicism, dup(22q), trisomy 22, and ring 21. There are also

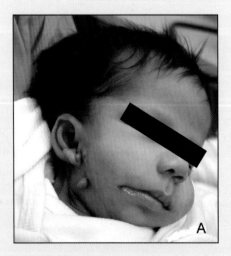
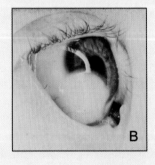

FIGURE 5–6. Oculoauriculovertebral spectrum. **A.** Note the right-sided hemifacial microsomia with preauricular ear tags, and macrostomia (large mouth that extends laterally). **B.** Epibulbar dermoid. This is a fleshy benign tumor on the conjunctiva that is common in this condition. (Courtesy Dr. Robert J. Shprintzen.)

instances in which oculoauriculovertebral spectrum can be seen in families, where it segregates as an autosomal dominant trait with variable expressivity. However, these cases are relatively uncommon, and are most often seen with less severe cases that are usually limited to the craniofacial region.

Several Mendelian syndromes can be mistaken for oculo-auriculovertebral spectrum, most notably Townes-Brock syndrome and branchial-oto-renal syndrome. Accurate diagnosis is important because each condition has different medical management issues as well as recurrence risks. Townes-Brock syndrome is characterized by imperforate anus, renal anomalies, triphalangeal thumbs, and other anomalies of the hands and feet, including fusion of metatarsals, absent bones, and supernumerary thumbs. Other features include mild sensorineural deafness, and lop ears. Branchial-oto-renal syndrome is characterized by renal anomalies, deafness, and congenital branchial cleft cysts. However, hemifacial microsomia, including preauricular skin tags, can be seen as well in both syndromes, which may cause them to be misdiagnosed as oculo-auriculovertebral spectrum. This can be a significant mistake, as both Townes Brock and branchio-oto-renal syndromes are inherited in an autosomal dominant manner, meaning the recurrence risk can be as high as 50% if one parent is affected) to less than 1% (if neither parent is affected). This is quite different for OAV, which has a 2 to 3% empiric recurrence risk. Therefore, careful clinical evaluation is warranted.

The diagnostic approach to malformations varies with the clinical pattern in which they are present. Although the genetic etiology of associations is by definition unknown and complex field defects are likely due to a single fetal vascular disruption episode, the likelihood of identifying an underlying cause is greater with sequences and syndromes but their etiology may be quite variable. Chromosomal abnormalities are one potential cause. Syndromes may also result from the complex interaction of multiple genes, multifactorial effects of genetic susceptibility under a necessary environmental influence, environmental factors such as teratogens or viral infections, or single gene defects alone. Single gene defects that result in congenital anomalies can follow any traditional Mendelian inheritance pattern, including autosomal dominant, autosomal recessive, or x-linked. It is also useful to consider nontraditional modes of genetic inheritance, such as mitochondrial gene mutations, imprinting errors or uniparental disomy, and triplet repeat expansion disease. Also, more than one distinct cause may potentially result in the same final malformation. Such is the case with a common malformation like micrognathia, where a small chin can be attributed to a collagen defect in Stickler syndrome or to a chromosomal deletion in velocardiofacial syndrome.

For many children with multiple congenital craniofacial anomalies, diagnosis of a genetic syndrome remains largely clinically based, thus relying on the ability of the clinician to correctly interpret and recognize patterns in physical findings, developmental delays, and family history. However, with the recent completion of sequencing of the human genome as part of the Human Genome Project, more genes are being identified that are causative of individual syndromes. This expanding knowledge base is rapidly increasing our ability to confirm clinically suspected diagnoses with specific genetic tests. Newer technology such as DNA microarrays are now clinically available, making it possible to simultaneously screen for hundreds of genetic errors associated with an entire category of disorders. Thus, it is worthwhile to consider revisiting the etiology of older patients with unknown or unconfirmed diagnoses every 3 to 5 years in an effort to clarify their prognosis, recurrence risk, and potentially even management decisions as the virtual explosion of genetic information unfolds.

REFERENCES

Lalani, S. R., Safiullah, A. M., Fernbach, S. D., Harutyunyan, K. G., Thaller C, Peterson, L. E., et al. (2006). Spectrum of CHD7 mutations in 110 individuals with CHARGE syndrome and genotype-phenotype correlation. *American Journal of Human Genetics*, *78*, 303–314.

Pagon, R. A., Graham, J. M., Jr., Zonana. J, & Young, S. L. (1981). Coloboma, congenital heart disease, and choanal atresia with multiple anomalies: CHARGE association. *Journal of Pediatrics*, *99*, 223–227.

Robin, N. H., Franklin, J., Prucka, S., Ryan, A. B., & Grant, J. H. (2005). Clefting, amniotic bands, and polydactyly: A distinct phenotype that supports an intrinsic mechanism for amniotic band sequence. *American Journal of Medical Genetics*, *137*, 298–301.

RECOMMENDED READING

Aase, J. M. (1990). *Diagnostic dysmorphology*. New York: Plenum.

Cohen, M. M. (1997). *The child with multiple birth defects* (2nd ed.). Cambridge: Oxford University Press.

Falk, M. J., & Robin, N. H. (2004). The primary care physician's approach to congenital anomalies. *Primary Care Clinical Office Practice*, *31*(3), 605–619.
A review that covers the topics discussed in this chapter.

Falk M. J., & Robin, N.H. (2005). The physical examination in clinical genetics. In M. J. Dunn, L. B. Jorde, P. F. R. Little, & S. Subramaniam (Eds.), *Encyclopedia of genetics, genomics, proteomics and bioinformatics* (chap. 99). Baltimore: Wiley.

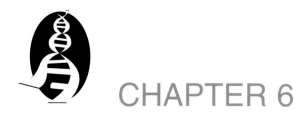

CHAPTER 6

Genetic Testing: Cytogenetics, Biochemical Genetics, and Molecular Genetics

EDWARD J. LOSE, M.D.
NATHANIEL H. ROBIN, M.D.

*T*his chapter provides an overview of the history, techniques, and interpretation of the three forms of genetic testing that are used in clinical practice: cytogenetics, DNA-based molecular testing, and biochemical analysis. Each is quite different in terms of the technology that is used and in what is actually being tested, but they are complementary. For that reason it is common that two or even all three would be employed as part of the evaluation of a patient.

By their nature, each type of genetic testing is complicated. It can be a challenge to explain this testing to patients and/or their families, why it is being done, what it will show, and what the limitations are. This is one of the major points covered in the genetic counseling process, which is covered in more detail in Chapters 7 and 8. Genetic testing not only is scientifically complex, but also brings up concerns that go beyond the medical issues. These include practical concerns, such as insurance discrimination, and ethical and legal questions. These are discussed in more detail in Chapter 7, but it is important to realize at the outset that these issues often are as important to patients as the medical information that genetic testing can provide. Because the primary care provider is often asked by patients and/or their parents about genetic testing—"What are they testing?" "What will it really tell us?" "Is it necessary?"—it is essential to have at least a rudimentary understanding of the various genetic tests.

AN OVERVIEW: THE DIFFERENCE BETWEEN CYTOGENETICS, MOLECULAR GENETICS, AND BIOCHEMICAL ANALYSIS

To patients, parents, and many health care providers, genetic testing is a mystery. Not only are they unfamiliar with the techniques of the various forms of testing, but they also often have a limited understanding of what is being tested and, perhaps most importantly, the limitations of these tests. When explaining genetic testing to patients and parents in clinical situations, it is useful to employ a simple analogy: an encyclopedia. Even in this age of computer-based databases, most people are familiar with the multiple volume encyclopedias in which each volume contained all topics that began with that letter (Figure 6-1).

As we tell our patients, our genes are the instruction manual to make the body, and they are arranged on chromosomes. Each chromosome is akin to a volume of the encyclopedia. Within each volume are chapters, pages, sentences, and words, just as each chromosome contains numerous genes. In this manner, chromosome analysis is as if we are looking at the outward appearance of the encyclopedia. We can see if one volume is missing a chapter, or has several chapters too many. Unfortunately, by looking from the outside we cannot tell if page 342 is missing in volume G, or if there is a typographical error in paragraph 2, page 277, volume M. Such alterations are analogous to smaller mutations within the genes. These are detectable only if you know where to look and open the book. Similarly, one can only detect a small genetic alteration such as a point mutation if you know what gene to test. This is akin to molecular DNA-based testing.

Chromosome Analysis

Although most people, the lay public, and health care professionals alike, think of genetic testing as a very recent technology, cytogenetic analysis entered clinical use in the early 1960s. This is still the most commonly ordered genetic test in the evaluation of children with developmental delay and/or congenital anomalies.

Chromosomes were originally discovered in the late 1800s. Several decades later, the chromosome was postulated to be the carrier of genetic traits, and several known inherited conditions were predicted to be caused by a change in the total number of chromosomes. Unfortunately, such theo-

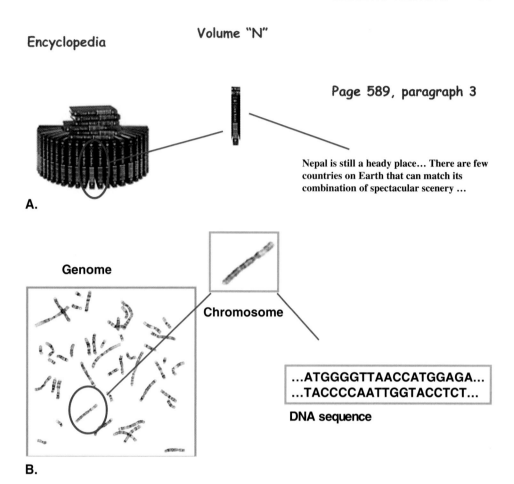

Encyclopedia

Volume "N"

Page 589, paragraph 3

Nepal is still a heady place... There are few
countries on Earth that can match its
combination of spectacular scenery ...

A.

Genome

Chromosome

...ATGGGGTTAACCATGGAGA...
...TACCCCAATTGGTACCTCT...

DNA sequence

B.

FIGURE 6–1. Comparison of information gathering from an encyclopedia (A) and cytogenetic testing and DNA-based molecular diagnosis testing (B).

ries could not be tested for many years, and it was not until the 1950s that it was first possible to separate chromosomes to permit accurate observation under the microscope. At this time, the normal number of human chromosomes was found to be 46, or 23 pairs (it had been thought to be 48 for many years). Individual chromosome pairs were "named," with the longest pair designated as "1," the shortest "22," with the 23rd pair being the sex chromosomes X and Y (Figure 6-2).

Almost immediately, many papers were published describing patients with well-known clinical conditions in which a change in the chromosome number was found. These include Down syndrome (three of chromosome 21 or trisomy 21), Edward syndrome (Trisomy 18), Patau syndrome (Trisomy 13), Klinefelter syndrome (XXY), and Turner syndrome (with only one X chromosome).

The next major breakthrough in chromosome technology came with the ability to "Band" chromosomes, giving them the characteristic black and white

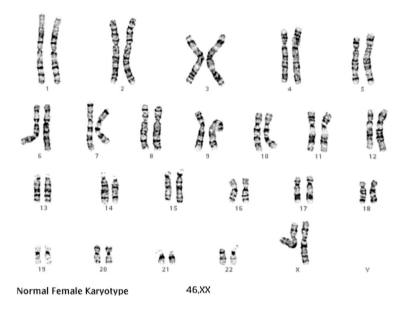

Normal Female Karyotype   46,XX

FIGURE 6–2. Normal female karyotype. Note the two copies of the "X" chromosome, no "Y" chromosome.

stripped banding pattern unique to each chromosome. This also ushered in a new level of chromosome nomenclature (see Chromosome Structure and Nomenclature). This not only made it possible to distinguish chromosomes of a similar size, it permitted the detection of small changes in a chromosome, such as duplications (an extra copy of material of a chromosome), deletions (missing a portion of a chromosome), insertions (material from one chromosome inserted into another), and translocations (swapped material between two chromosomes). Over time, it became possible to "stretch out" the chromosomes, enhancing the detail of the banding patterns, which then permits identification of even smaller missing or extra pieces. This is the basic chromosome analysis that is still performed in clinical cytogenetics labs today. However, by using the naked eye, the size of a detectable missing or extra piece is still relatively large, 5 to 10 million base pairs, thus the need for other techniques, such as fluorescence in-situ hybridization, or as it is more commonly known, "FISH."

Chromosome Structure and Nomenclature

Chromosomes share a common general structure (Figure 6–3). Each chromosome has a section called a centromere, which appears as a pinched-in section. This structure is important in the pairing and replication of the chromosomes during cell division (see Shaffer & Tommerup [2005] for a complete discussion of cell cycle, chromosome replication, and cell division). The centromere divides each chromosome into two halves, or "arms." The shorter arm is designated "p," for the French word *petit*, meaning "small." The longer arm is designated "q," which was chosen because it followed "p."

The advent of banding also brought a new level of nomenclature to chromosomes, as each dark band had a designation. Closest to the centromere was band "1," the next band "2," and so on until the telomere, which is the name of the end of the chromosome. With time, as chromosomes were able to be "stretched," it became apparent that many single dark bands, in fact, contained multiple light and dark segments within them. These subbands were designated by a second number (e.g., "11," or "12." Now banding is so fine that bands are designated to a second decimal point (e.g., "12.22").

One last and very important point is pronunciation. Geneticists pronounce "15q11.22" as "fifteen q one-one point two-two," not "fifteen q eleven twenty-two." Say it in the former manner and you will be recognized as someone who knows genetics. Say it in the latter and face ridicule. However, this seemingly complex nomenclature is not used to merely confuse the uninitiated. It has permitted a standardized system that is used to describe chromosomal abnormalities. This system is far too complex to review here. The interested reader is referred to Shaffer and Tommerup (2005).

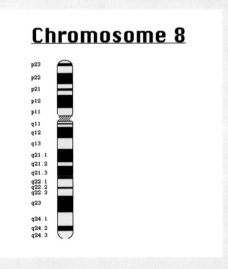

FIGURE 6–3. An ideogram of chromosome 8 showing the named bands. From http://wimp.nsm.uh.edu/chromo8.gif

How Is a Chromosome Analysis Done?

Chromosomes must be obtained from dividing cells from the patient. The most common source is blood or, more specifically, white blood cells. Red blood cells and platelets are the only cells that do not have nuclei, and therefore do not have DNA. All other cells in the body contain the entire complement of an individual's genes.

The patient's blood is placed in a culture that contains a chemical (phytohemagglutinin) that stimulates the division of the T lymphocytes. After 3 days, another chemical is added (colchicine) that stops cell division at metaphase, the point at which the chromosomes are most condensed, and therefore able to be studied. The cells then are treated with a hypotonic salt solution and fixed with a methanol/acetic acid mixture. Drops from the solution containing the fixed cells are dropped on a microscope slide, where they rupture and spill out the chromosomes. The slide is banded with trypsin and stained with Giemsa stain. A cytogenetic technician then counts and analyzes the chromosomes, making sure there is the correct number, and each chromosome is morphologically normal. After a review by the laboratory's medical director, the final report is generated and the karyotype described using standardized nomenclature (see The Building Blocks of Genes and Chromosomes).

Fluorescence in situ Hybridization (FISH)

FISH is used to detect missing or extrachromosomal segments that are smaller than can be detected using Giemsa-banded chromosome analysis. Unlike standardized cytogenetic analysis, when ordering a FISH test, one must have a suspicion as to the specific abnormality, as FISH uses a probe to look for the presence of a specific genetic segment.

FISH probes are constructed after a lab finds that a syndrome is caused by a deletion of a specific genetic region. A well-known example is Velocardiofacial syndrome (VCFS, see Chapter 11 for more details on VCFS), which is caused by a microdeletion on chromosome 22 band q11.2. This deletion typically is too small to be seen on routine chromosome analysis. However, a FISH probe can be used to visualize the VCFS region. In someone who has VCFS, only one chromosome 22 will show a signal, as the other is missing the region to which the fluorescent probe hybridizes. If the person does not have the condition, both chromosomes 22 will show the signal, each with an intact VCFS region (Figure 6–4A–D). Many other syndromes are diagnosed by FISH, including Williams syndrome and Prader-Willi syndrome.

One relatively new application of FISH technology is **subtelomere analysis**. Telomeres are the ends of chromosomes. The region just proximal to the telomere (closer to the centromere) is particularly gene-rich, meaning it contains a larger percentage of genes than other parts of the chromosome, and

The Building Blocks of Genes and Chromosomes

Deoxyribonucleic acid, known as its shorthand DNA, is the molecule used to encode our genetic information. It does so using a specific sequence of 4 chemical bases: guanine (G), cytosine (C), adenine (A) and thymidine (T). These bases are bonded to each other in a linear fashion called a strand. Each strand is 'read' in groups of three called codons. Each codon is a code for a specific amino acid. There are 20 amino acids, and these are the building blocks of the proteins found in the human body. One may ask why DNA is an acid, but made of bases. The bases on the strand are attached to each other with sugars and an acidic phosphate making the whole strand an acid.

Each strand bonds weakly to an opposite strand in a very specific fashion: A bonds to T and G bonds to C. Together, these form the well-known double helix DNA molecule that was first discovered in the mid-1950s.

Although a chromosome contains DNA, it also has many other associated proteins that are involved in the folding and maintenance of the chromosome structure; and regulation of which genes are expressed. Histones are proteins that support the scaffold to which the DNA double helix attaches in a coil. The histones detach and expose the gene that needs to be used. Other proteins are used to turn genes off or on by binding to the starting segment called the promoter.

The proteins are not made directly from the DNA codon. Another molecule called ribonucleic acid or RNA reads the codon off the DNA template. A third molecule called transfer RNA or tRNA brings the amino acids and places them in the exact order specified by RNA.

This is of course a very quick overview of the basic science of DNA structure, replication, and translation. There are many excellent texts that review it in much more detail, several which are listed at the end of the chapter under Recommended Reading.

is known as the "subtelomere."[1] Subtelomere analysis is a test that uses a FISH probe unique to each chromosome's subtelomere region to look for a deletion and/or duplication that is not visible using Giemsa-banded chromosome analysis. Subtelomere abnormalities are found in about 6% of children with severe

---

[1]Several important facts about the relationship of genes and chromosomes: (1) More than 80% of the DNA in the human genome does not code for genes. These sequences, often called "junk DNA," have no known function. (2) Genes are not evenly distributed among all chromosomes. Some chromosomes have a much higher number of genes in proportion to their size

Florescence *in-situ* hybridization

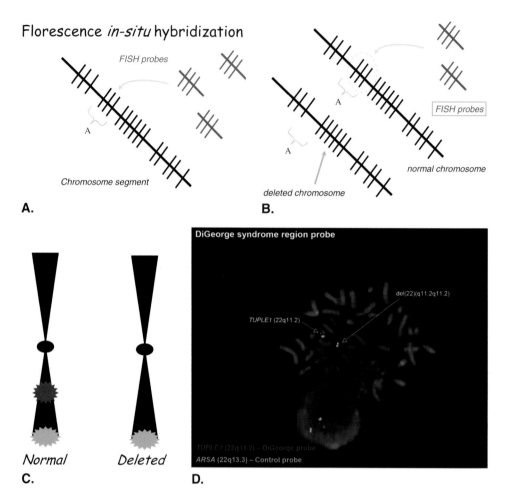

A. **B.**

C. **D.**

FIGURE 6–4. A. FISH probes are developed that bind to a particular part of the genome ("A"). Previously, researchers have shown that patients missing "A" have a genetic syndrome. **B.** The FISH probes bind to the normal chromosome with the intact "A" segment, but cannot bind to the chromosome with the deleted "A" segment. **C.** The normal chromosome has the red signal, showing the disease-associated segment is present. The deleted chromosome does not have the signal, and therefore is deleted for the segment. The green signals are used both as controls and to identify the chromosome. As is evident in D, chromosomes undergoing FISH lose their identifying characteristics. **D.** An actual FISH test. The red signal is the probe for the region that is deleted in patients with Williams syndrome. The green is the control for chromosome 22, the location of the velocardiofacial syndrome segment. One of this patient's chromosome 22 do not bind the velocardiofacial syndrome probe. They are said to be deleted, which confirms the diagnosis of Velocardiofacial syndrome.

than others. For example, chromosome 22 is particularly gene rich, whereas chromosome 13 is fairly gene poor. (3) Genes also are not evenly distributed along each chromosome. The ends of each chromosome are especially rich in genes compared to the rest of the chromosome.

idiopathic mental retardation. They are especially useful to order if there is a family history of unexplained developmental problems, and if the patient has congenital anomalies that do not comprise a recognizable syndrome.

Molecular Genetic (DNA-Based) Testing

Using an earlier analogy, DNA-based testing is the search for misspelled words among the volumes in our genetic encyclopedia. Unlike cytogenetic testing, where no prior suspicion of a particular location is required, finding an error in the DNA sequence requires that we know where to look (e.g., which gene or genes to test). Often, even that may not be enough, as single base pair mutations[2] may be in parts of the gene that are, for technical reasons, difficult or impossible to detect. Or, as in the case with deafness and many other genetically determined disorders, genetic or even etiologic heterogeneity may be present. *Genetic heterogeneity* is the recognition that a mutation in two or more different genes can cause the same phenotype. *Etiologic heterogeneity* is the finding that there are genetic and nongenetic causes of a particular phenotype. Perhaps the best example of this is hearing impairment. Not only are more than 100 different genes estimated to be involved in hearing impairment, but there are many nongenetic causes as well, such as congenital infection, noise exposure, and drugs/toxins. For example, mutations in the *gap junction beta 2* (*GJβ2*) gene are the most common form of genetic deafness, being found in about 30% of deaf infants. One could test *GJβ2* in a deaf child and receive a negative result. There are several reasons for this outcome. It is possible that the child's deafness is indeed genetic, but caused by mutations in another gene. Alternatively, it is possible that the child's deafness is not genetic, but caused by a prenatal cytomegalovirus infection. Finally, and most confusing, it is possible that the child's deafness is due to *GJβ2* mutations, but they are in a region of the gene that was not tested due to technical reasons. These issues are discussed in more detail in Chapters 7, 8, and 10.

Unlike cytogenetic testing, DNA-based testing can use a nonliving sample from the patient. Any cell that has DNA can be used, but blood (white blood cells) is the most common source. Other material is often used includes amniocytes obtained for prenatal diagnosis, cheek brush samples, skin biopsy, and even tissue embedded in paraffin blocks from surgical specimens or autopsies (note: due to technical reasons, not all DNA tests can use all materials).

---

[2]Proteins are made of chemicals called amino acids. The amino acid sequences of many proteins have been known for decades. The DNA molecule contains the instructions the cell uses in several steps to assemble proteins. Scientists worked backward and discovered the specific DNA sequences which produce these proteins. Additional clues such as changes in chromosomes and sequences in lower animals (fruit flies, bacteria, yeast, mice, etc.) resulted in testing for the changes (mutations) in the gene sequence responsible for a syndrome.

Once the gene or genes to be tested are chosen, and DNA is obtained from the patient, the exact type of testing that will be performed is very variable. A comprehensive discussion is beyond the scope of this book, but suffice it to say that this is a fast changing field, with dozens of sophisticated techniques used in molecular DNA-based diagnosis.

The many different techniques are needed, as there are many forms of gene mutations (Figure 6–5A and 6–5B). These include point mutations, small deletions, translocations, trinucleotide repeats, and methylation abnormalities. Some DNA sequence differences between individuals and ethnic groups are common and do not result in disease. These benign changes are called **polymorphisms**. Other changes may lead to a change in the amino acid sequence of the protein, but result in no change in the function of the protein. These are called a **conservative change** and are not thought to cause disease. Other changes cause the function of the protein to be disrupted. Such changes are disease-causing, and are called **mutations**.

A **point mutation** is a change in a single DNA base pair. This can lead to a protein with a different amino acid composition at a given location, with the new amino acid deleteriously altering the function of the protein. The best example is sickle cell disease, where a single base pair change in the sixth codon of the beta globin gene produces a different and abnormally functioning hemoglobin. Point mutations can also result in a truncated (smaller) protein. A **small deletion** can lead to the production of a truncated protein, or it can cause the protein not to be made at all.

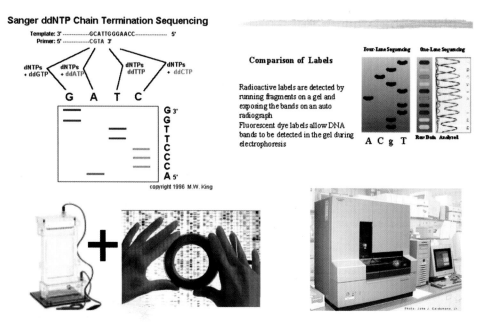

FIGURE 6–5. DNA gene sequencing. (Reproduced with permission of Dr. Michael W. King from http://jsu.indstate.edu/mwking)

Many labs in the United States offer DNA-based testing. A fairly complete list can be found at http://www.genetests.org/. This Web site lists the labs that offer testing for various conditions, but it is very useful as they are catalogued by the condition. Not all labs are the same, either. Some are large and offer testing for a long list of diseases; others are smaller and offer testing for only a few select few disorders. Often, testing for a particular disease is offered in several labs, especially if it is a common disorder. However, it is important to recognize that different labs may utilize different techniques in testing the same gene. In some cases, this may not really matter, as each technique is equally valid; in other cases, one technique is far superior to the other. Making that determination is often very difficult, and typically requires an advanced understanding of the techniques and disease. In most cases, it is most efficient and beneficial to the patient and family if decisions on genetic testing were made after consultation with a clinical geneticist or genetic counselor. Chapters 7 and 8 discuss the complexities of genetic testing in more detail.

Molecular DNA-based genetic testing is most often ordered to confirm a suspected diagnosis of a genetic disorder. For example, a patient with deafness and vision loss may be suspected to have Usher syndrome. Genetic testing can be ordered to confirm that, and to define which type and identify the inheritance pattern—autosomal recessive, autosomal dominant, or X-linked. Molecular testing may also be ordered for carrier testing. For example, if the patient with Usher syndrome is found to have autosomal recessive Usher syndrome due to mutation in the gene, their normal-hearing sibling may wish to know if he or she carries one copy of the Usher gene, and is, therefore, at risk of having an affected child.

Array Comparative Genomic Hybridization

Array comparative genomic hybridization (CGH) is a new technology that represents a fusion of cytogenetic and molecular genetic testing. Its purpose is to identify DNA copy number variations (gains or losses of genetic material) that are too small to be detected by Giemsa-banded chromosome analysis and too large to be found by most molecular techniques. It involves hybridization of patient and reference DNA (each labeled with a different fluorophore) onto DNA probes bound to a glass slide. Following hybridization and washing to remove unbound DNA, the relative levels of fluorescence are measured using a special laser scanner and computer software to generate the final graphical plots. The probes are usually genomic clones and can be chosen to represent either the whole genome or only target areas of the genome known to be associated with specific syndromes due to recurrent gains (duplications) or losses (deletions) (Figure 6-6). The advantage of array CGH over FISH is that it can test hundreds of genomic regions for small duplications and/or deletions in just one experiment.

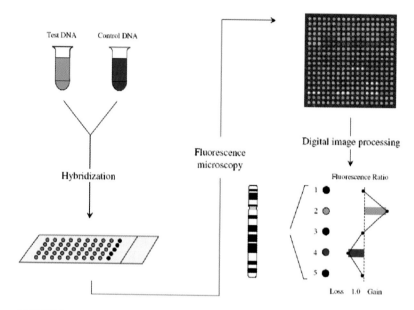

FIGURE 6–6. Complementary genomic hybridization or CGH allows the simultaneous detection of missing or extra pieces of a person's chromosome. Small pieces of human DNA are placed or 'written' on the slide. The patient's DNA is cut into small pieces and a fluorescent molecule is attached to each. The patient's DNA is then placed on the slide and the small fragments find the complementary strand on the slide and bind. Light is shined on the slide and where the patient's DNA binds to the slide DNA is lit a certain color. A detector "reads" the glowing circles and a computer lists what pieces of the patient's DNA match the control human DNA. (Diagram courtesy of Dr. Fady Mikhail, University of Alabama-Birmingham, Department of Genetics.)

CHIP TECHNOLOGY

With technology similar to that used in CGH, it will soon be possible to set up a test that can test multiple genes simultaneously. Such DNA "chips" will have the genetic sequence of dozens of genes. This would have immediate impact on patients with hearing impairment. Today, genetic testing for patients with hearing impairment requires testing individual genes sequentially. This is not possible, as it is far too costly and inefficient. Using this new technology, a single chip can test several dozen hearing impairment-related genes simultaneously. Although this technology is not yet available, it will be in the not too distant future.

Biochemical Testing

Biochemical testing, unlike cytogenetics and molecular testing, does not directly analyze DNA. Rather, it looks at chemical compounds that are the products of our cellular metabolism, the various pathways that provide us energy, as well as the building blocks of our cells. These chemical compounds are made as the end result of biochemical pathways that are made up of substrates, enzymes and cofactors, and products. Cofactors are additional chemicals required to make an enzyme function properly and are more commonly referred to as vitamins. Enzymes catalyze reactions in which a substance is converted into a product. If there is a block in one step, due to a missing or poorly functional enzyme or cofactor, abnormal chemicals back up and accumulate in the tissues, blood, and urine. The resulting conditions are called inherited disorder of metabolism, sometimes referred to as inborn errors of metabolism or just metabolic diseases.

Although some metabolic diseases do have hearing impairment as one component manifestation (Table 6–1), we have spent very little space in this book reviewing them. Many metabolic diseases present in infancy in otherwise normal-appearing children. Common signs and symptoms of these early onset metabolic diseases include progressive lethargy, poor feeding, and an abnormal breathing pattern. Others present later in life, and can have associated dysmorphic findings, developmental delay, or significant neuromuscular problems. Recurrent bouts of severe illness are another common finding.

These findings are very nonspecific, meaning they also can be caused by any number of other medical problems. Confirmation of the diagnosis of a metabolic disease requires identification of an abnormal biochemical profile in the patient's blood, urine, or spinal fluid. Although this will point to the correct diagnosis, confirmation often requires demonstration of the enzyme deficiency. In some instances, this can be done in blood testing, but some disorders require testing skin, muscle, or other cells. For many conditions, the gene that codes for the abnormal enzyme is known and can, therefore, be directly tested by molecular techniques.

NEWBORN SCREENING

For many metabolic diseases, early therapy is a key to avoiding significant problems; for this reason, most states now utilize expanded screening of the blood of newborns to identify a wide range of inherited disorders. This expanded screen tests for compounds that accumulate if an enzyme is deficient. For some disorders, it actually tests the enzyme level in the baby's blood (biotinidase). The hope is to diagnose early and institute therapy—often as simple as a change in diet. One such example is phenylketonuria (PKU).

TABLE 6–1. Metabolic Disease That Feature Hearing Impairment as One Finding

Age of Detection	Main Symptoms	Disorders

Neonatal to early infancy	Dysmorphism
	  Severe mental retardation
	  Hypotonia
	  Retinitis pigmentosa
	  Seizures
	Congenital encephalopathy
	  Episodes of coma
	All of the above plus
	intracranial calcifications
		Zellweger syndrome and variants
		Rhizomelic chondrodysplasia punctata
		Acyl CoA oxidase deficiency
		Hyperkynureninuria
		
		Cockayne syndrome
		Alport syndrome

Late infancy to early childhood	Failure to thrive
	  Hepatomegaly
	  Diarrhea
	  Osteoporosis
	  Retinitis pigmentosa
	Gout
	  Arthritis
	  Hyperuricemia
	  Ataxia
	  Hypotonia
	  Psychotic behavior
	Coarse facies
	  Dysostosis multiplex
	
	Alopecia
	  Cutaneous rashes
	  Hypotonia, coma
	  Lactic acidosis
	Megaloblastic anemia
	  Diabetes
	  Responsiveness to
	  thiamine
	Ichthyosis
	  Hepatomegaly
	  Myopathy
	  Vacuolated lymphocytes
	Lactic acidosis
	  Short stature
	  Dementia
	  Weakness
	  Ragged-red fibers
	  Multiorgan failure
	  Strokes
		Infantile Refsum disease
		
		PRPP synthetase overactivity
		
		Mucopolysaccharidoses types I, II, IV
		Mannosidosis (alpha and beta)
		Mucolipidosis type II
		
		Biotinidase deficiency (biotin responsive)
		
		Megaloblastic anemia, thiamine responsive
		Wolfram syndrome
		
		Neutral lipid storage disorder
		
		Mitochondrial encephalomyopathy MELAS, MERRF, and Kearns-Sayre syndromes due to various respiratory chain errors (nuclear mitochondrial gene deletions or insertions)

TABLE 6–1. *(continued)*

Age of Detection	Main Symptoms	Disorders
Late childhood to adolescence and adulthood	Mental retardation Retinitis pigmentosa	Infantile Refsum disease Usher syndrome type II

	Ataxia
	   Peripheral neuropathy
	   Retinitis pigmentosa
	   Ichthyosis
	   Anosmia	

	Ptosis
	   Ophthalmoplegia
	   Retinitis pigmentosa
	   Myopathy
	   Atrioventricular
	   dissociation
	   Hyperlactacidemia
		Kearns-Sayre syndrome (mitochondrial DNA deletion) and other respiratory chain disorders.

	Myocionic epilepsy
	   Ragged red fibers
	   Ataxia
		MERRF syndrome (mitochondrial tRNA Lys mutation)

	Angiokeratoma Mental retardation	β-Mannosidosis

Source: Reprinted with permission from: *The Metabolic and Molecular Basis of Inherited Disease* (8th ed., p. 6295) by C. R. Scriver, A. L. Beaudet, W. S. Sly, and D. Valle (Eds.), 2001. Copyright McGraw-Hill 2001.

This was among the first diseases to be tested for on the newborn screen. PKU is an inherited disorder of metabolism in which the enzyme that converts phenylalanine to tyrosine is deficient, so phenylalanine accumulates in the baby's blood. At high levels, phenylalanine is toxic to the brain. When PKU is identified, the infant is put on a diet reduced in the amino acid phenylalanine, and blood phenylalanine levels decrease to appropriate treatment levels. The enzymatic chain of reactions changing phenylalanine to tyrosine is deprived of the starting amino acid, so the toxic chemicals are reduced.

An example of a metabolic disease with hearing loss is biotinidase deficiency. The vitamin biotin is used by many different enzymes (called carboxylases) as a cofactor. Biotinidase is the enzyme that recycles biotin so that the body can use is repeatedly. When the body is unable to recycle and reuse biotin because of a deficiency of biotinidase, the enzymes for which biotin is a cofactor do not work efficiently. As a result of this, abnormal chemicals are excreted in the urine. Untreated biotinidase deficiency results in sensorineural hearing loss, optic atrophy, lethargy, diffuse brain damage, and a severe dermatitis rash. Treatment with simple oral biotin may promptly result in clinical improvement. Most states now test for biotin deficiency in the newborn screening programs.

Newborn screening has revolutionized the diagnosis and treatment of metabolic diseases. Many children are now diagnosed immediately after birth and begun on therapy, before the onset of symptoms. Furthermore, as technology has advanced, the number of diseases that can be screened has increased dramatically, the so-called "expanded newborn screen." Most states have a biochemical geneticist specializing in this group of diseases. When a baby's screen is abnormal, the infant's pediatrician and the biochemical geneticist are notified by the state newborn screening program so that therapy can be instituted and follow-up testing performed. One important aspect to recognize with newborn screening is that there is a wide range of enzyme activity in the normal population, so there is an overlap of normal chemical profiles with the abnormal range. Therefore, many infants who have an abnormality detected on the newborn screen are, in fact, normal. The newborn screen is a *screening* test, designed not to miss any affected children even though it will falsely label many samples as abnormal (so-called "false positives"). The pediatrician and biochemical geneticist will arrange further diagnostic testing to determine if the child is truly affected. These diagnostic tests look at the pattern of chemical compounds in blood, urine, and occasionally cerebrospinal fluid to determine if there is a normal pattern of chemical compounds, or an abnormal pattern that might indicate a metabolic disease.

RECOMMENDED READING

Cogan, J. D., & Phillips, J. A. III. (2006). New methods in genetic diagnosis including prenatal diagnosis. *Pediatric Endocrinology Reviews, 3*(Suppl. 3), 424–433.

Haley, R. S., & Mori, C. A. (1999). *The human genome: A user's guide.* San Diego, CA: Academic Press.

Hartwell, L., Hood, L., Goldbert, M., Reynolds, L., & Veres, R. (Eds.). (2008). *Genetics: From genes to genomes* (3rd ed.). New York: McGraw-Hill.

Korf, B. R. (2006). *Human genetics and genomics* (3rd ed.). London: Blackwell.

Shaffer, L. G., & Tommerup, N. (Eds.). (2005). *An international system for human cytogenetic nomenclature.* Basel, Switzerland: S. Karger.

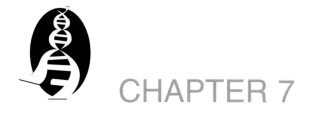

CHAPTER 7

Ethical Issues in Genetic Testing

INTRODUCTION

Advances in genetics have promised many benefits to individuals and society. Although, in general, the public has viewed genetic advances favorably, concerns about how this information will be used have been raised. These concerns were recognized when the United States government initiated the Human Genome Project (HGP), as one integral component of this effort was the creation of a section to fund research and education on ethical, legal, and social implications (ELSI) of the effects of these genetic advances on individuals and on society. By no means are all the ethical issues relevant to medical genetics addressed in this chapter. Rather, this chapter is intended to provide a brief overview of bioethics, and how its principles relate to medical genetics.

A BRIEF HISTORY OF MEDICAL ETHICS

Although recognition of bioethics as medical discipline is relatively new, the notion of ethical standards in medical practice in Western culture can be traced to Hippocrates in the 5th century BC. The Hippocratic oath maintains that a physician should do no harm, respect his patient's privacy, and strive to do the best for his patient. These tenets can be found today in the core principals of modern bioethics (Table 7-1). Subsequent works such as "Medical Ethics," written in 1803 by English physician Thomas Pickering, the 1847 ethical code of the American Medical Association, and Dr. Richard Cabot emphasized

TABLE 7–1. Principles of Bioethics. The bioethical principles can provide a framework when discussing the ethics of a specific case or issue. However, they can never be viewed in isolation, but must always be balanced against each other in ethical decision making.

Autonomy:	The notion that an individual has the right to make their own medical decisions, free of coercion.
Beneficence:	The duty to assist another actively and directly, with a minimum possibility of causing harm.
Nonmaleficence:	Simply put, this means to do no harm. This includes not only active and intentional harm, which is always prohibited, but also it is meant to limit the possibility of unintentional harm in the course of trying to help.
Justice (societal and political):	This is the concept of fairness, that each person is entitled to equal medical care. This can come into conflict with the notion that health care is a finite resource, and some limits must be placed on its allocation.

Note: For further information, including illustrative cases, please see http://depts.washington.edu/bioethx/tools/princpl.html#prin4

societal concerns as well as responsibility to an individual patient. However, it was not until the Nuremberg Code of 1946 that a strict ethical code for research was established. Created in response to the atrocities in human experimentation performed in Nazi Germany during World War II, the outlined principles addressed the need to protect research subjects from excessive risk, regardless of the potential perceived benefit from the proposed research. From this came the concepts of informed consent and the notion of institutional review boards as the monitoring mechanism of research.

PRINCIPLES OF BIOETHICS

The four basic principles listed in Table 7-1 are commonly cited as the underpinnings of modern bioethics. Each has origins in the teachings of ethicists dating back to Socrates, Plato, and Aristotle, and includes Immanuel Kant, Thomas Hobbs, John Rawls, Jeremy Betham, and Stuart Mill, as well as the three dominant Western religions, Judaism, Christianity, and Islam. Making ethically sound decisions involves balancing these four principles, as they often are at odds in a given situation. Furthermore, although these are considered the four fundamental principles for bioethical reasoning, they are by no means an all-inclusive list of issues that are to be considered.

Autonomy refers to an individual's right to make his or her own decisions based on his or her own free will, be it to choose whether or not to have children, move to the city or a farm, or refuse medical treatment. This individual freedom of choice is a basic right in any democratic society, and should not be challenged unless that choice harms others. Autonomy evolved as a driving principle of bioethics during the 1960s in conjunction with the societal push toward individuality and freedom to choose. In this regard, autonomy was a rejection of paternalism, the notion of the venerable wise physician making decisions for his patients because he knew what was best for the patient better than the patient did. Autonomy rejects that argument, mandating that it is the patient's right to decide what he or she wants regarding treatments or evaluations. Patient autonomy is among the most cherished values for genetics professionals, and represents the basis for the core principle of genetics: "nondirective" counseling.

Autonomy was once considered by some bioethicists the most important of principles to consider when deciding ethical dilemmas, but it is now recognized that other principles must be considered as well and given equal weight.

Beneficence refers to the desire to help our fellow man. It is a very old value, as it can be found in Judeo-Christian-Muslim teachings of charity toward our fellow man. For physicians, beneficence is both a value to strive toward as well as a duty, as it is expected that physicians will act in the patient's best interest and not be motivated by greed or other less noble motives. Beneficence can come into conflict with autonomy when an individual exercises his or her free choice and chooses not to be helped, such as when an individual declines genetic testing even when it might identify if she is at increased risk for developing breast cancer. Beneficence implies that we should convince the person to have the testing, as it has obvious benefits for that person's health. But, as dictated by autonomy, it is that person's right to decline testing. That is why genetic counseling is nondirective, and does not push a patient toward a specific decision.

Nonmaleficence, the desire to do no harm, draws directly from the Hippocratic oath. It is better to do nothing than to actively harm a patient. As in the example above, we want our patient to have genetic testing for cancer susceptibility because it will greatly enhance her health care (beneficence), it is her right to decline it (autonomy), and we should not try to coerce her (nonmaleficence). Similarly, in instances where testing an adult child may reveal that the parent has the same disease, the parents may not want to know if they carry the deleterious gene, but the adult child does. Do the adult child's right to know (autonomy) and medical benefit (beneficence) outweigh harm to the parents (nonmaleficence)?

Justice really has two components, individual and societal. Individual justice refers to the basic belief that all people with a given disease should be treated equally, regardless of insurance coverage or social status. Societal justice refers to the larger issues regarding allocation of scarce resources. This has special relevance for genetics because genetic evaluations, testing, and treatments are very expensive, and not universally covered by insurance carriers.

STEPS IN ETHICAL REASONING

There are several discrete steps to take when confronting an ethical dilemma (Table 7–2). First, define the problem: identify what ethical principles, listed in Table 7–1, are in conflict. Although this may seem straightforward, it is often quite challenging, especially in clinical bioethics consultations. In clinical situations, the ethical issues are easily confused with other questions, such as those pertaining to medical management, law, or social situations.

The second step is to determine the facts and/or assumptions; the third to list potential alternatives or options; and the fourth to evaluate the possible choices or decisions that can be made, and how well each is justified based on ethical theory and principles.

Take, for example, a 22-year-old woman whose two maternal aunts and maternal grandmother each developed medullary thyroid carcinoma (MTC) in their 30s. A mutation in the RET gene, known to cause of MTC, was identified in one of the aunts, and this woman wishes to know if she is a carrier as well. Her mother, who has no cancer history, does not wish to be tested, as she does not want to know if she is at risk. Her daughter says that she is scared that she will have to have her thyroid removed if she is positive, and that she would feel very guilty if she had passed on this fate to her only daughter. However, in this case, a positive test in the 22-year-old is a de facto test for the mother as well, as it will mean that the mother is also a carrier. Should the 22-year-old be allowed to have testing, even though it may be testing her mother against her wishes?

1. *Define the problem by what ethical principals are in conflict:* The patient's autonomy (her desire to have herself tested), and a desire to help her (beneficence), as genetic testing will allow her to make medical management decisions to positively influence her health. The conflict arises in the desire not to harm her mother by forcing her to learn her genetic status (nonmalefiscence).

2. *Determine the facts and/or assumptions:* The *facts* include that this family does segregate a RET mutation, and testing this woman is medically appropriate. A positive result will allow her to make decisions to benefit

Table 7–2. Steps in Ethical Reasoning

1. Define the problem in terms of which ethical principals are in conflict.

2. Determine the facts and/or assumptions of the situation.

3. List potential alternatives or options.

4. Evaluate how well possible solutions are supported by ethical principles.

her care, as negative result will mean that she is not at elevated risk for developing cancer. Furthermore, only a positive result will be informative for the mother. If her daughter tests negative, it is not known if her mother is also negative, or if she is a carrier and did not pass on the mutant gene to her daughter. However, there are many assumptions here. Our patient's mother holds many misunderstandings about what a positive result will mean—it will not mean that she has to have her thyroid removed. Also, potential guilt seems to be an issue.

3. *List potential alternatives/options*: It is possible that, if these misconceptions and issues could be discussed with a medical professional, the mother might not maintain her reluctance to know her genetic status. Testing for the daughter could then proceed without ethical conflict. Alternatively, the daughter could be tested with the understanding that the results be kept from her mother. Although possible, this is not practical. Finally, the daughter could be denied testing due to the concerns of violating the mother's right not to know.

4. *Evaluate how well possible solutions are supported by ethical principles*: Testing the daughter regardless of the mother's concerns is supported by the notion of autonomy, especially when it is considered by many the primary ethical principle. Denying the daughter testing due to the mother's concerns would violate that primary concern.

Deciding the ethics of a case is not the same as deciding the outcome. Ethics committees make recommendations, which may or may not be followed by the parties involved. Furthermore, ethical decisions are made independent of other concerns, such as existing laws and hospital policies. Often these other concerns dictate the outcome of a given case, even if they conflict with the ethical decision.

GENETIC EXCEPTIONALISM

With the explosion of genetic information in the last 20 years has come many ethical questions, and among the most intriguing is "genetic exceptionalism," the notion that genetic information is so different from other medical information that it should be dealt with in a special manner. To some extent, the debate is moot, as genetic information already has taken a special place within all aspects of society, including medicine, law, and popular culture. Special laws have been passed in many states that provides limited protection against discrimination based on genetic test results, and similar federal legislation is currently being considered by the United States Congress. These laws and legislation are above and beyond existing laws for other forms of medical information and, therefore, serve to further emphasize the distinctiveness of genetic information from other medical information. However, is this distinction really valid? Is genetic information really so special that current medical privacy laws and other protections are inadequate in protecting it from being wrongfully used? Is it possible that this special attention is, in fact, detrimental?

The concept of genetic exceptionalism centers on several features about genetic information, features that some argue make genetic information unique among medical information: it is a predictive diary; it divulges information about family members; genetic information has been used to discriminate and stigmatize; and uncovering genetic risk may cause serious psychological harm. However, many authors have challenged these points, suggesting that, although very powerful, genetic information is not so distinct, and there is no clear justification to separate genetic information from other forms of medical information.

It is a predictive diary. Genetic test results can be used to make a diagnosis, such as chromosome analysis confirming the clinical diagnosis of Down syndrome. However, it is predictive genetic testing that has sparked the most debate. These tests have been described as a crystal ball through which we can see into our medical futures. Such images convey a certainty with a genetic test result that may be unfounded, but also is really no different than many other medical tests. For a genetic syndrome such as velocardiofacial syndrome (VCFS), identification of the genetic mutation (a submicroscopic deletion on chromosome 22, at band q11.22) confirms the diagnosis, and with it a very high risk for that child of having various medical complications, including immune deficiencies, endocrine dysfunction, learning disabilities, and psychiatric illness, such as depression and schizophrenia. Armed with this knowledge, steps can be taken to avoid or limit the impact of these associated problems. However, such complications can be addressed with frequent testing and evaluations. For example, a low TSH level may indicate incipient hypothyroidism disease. In this manner, genetic test results are really no different than other medical information. Similarly, high cholesterol and elevated blood pressure are tests that are used to predict coronary artery disease (CAD), and HIV testing is used to predict the development of AIDS. So the fact that it is predictive is not a distinguishing feature for genetic testing. Cholesterol and blood pressure are relatively weak predictors of CAD, whereas identifying a chromosome 22q11 deletion is a much stronger predictor for learning problems, and so on that are associated with VCFS. So, in this example, genetic testing will provide many benefits that other tests may not. It is not qualitatively different. They are all predictive tests. Genetic testing is just better.

Although both genetic and nongenetic tests can be strong or weak predictors for disease, there is another key difference—that of perception. Unlike a virus, a cholesterol level, or even a biopsy looking for cancer, most people perceive genetic information as internal, a part of themselves. Such feelings were echoed when President Clinton, at the announcement of the first draft of the Human Genome Project, referred to genes and "the language in which God created man." In this manner, many people view carrying a genetic mutation as an indication of an inherent and fundamental flaw in them, far different than external agents of disease. This reason may be at the core of why society views genetic information as different.

Genetic test results divulge information about family members. When testing an individual for a genetic mutation, one is, in fact, often testing their entire family. Identifying a mutation in a deafness-related gene means that the patient's relatives are also at risk. However, this is true for nongenetic tests as well. A diagnosis of a sexually transmitted disease such as HSV or HIV has important implications for that person's partners; a positive tuberculosis test means that this person's family members as well as other close contacts are at risk. What is different about genetic testing is that the risk is conferred only to biologically related individuals; for infectious diseases the risk extends to nonrelated social contacts. So, for genetic disease, genetic status can often be inferred based on the person's position in a pedigree, with the greater risk in those more closely related to the patient. It is, of course, best for the patient to inform his or her relatives of this risk, but occasionally the patient refuses. In such cases, what responsibility does the physician have to those at-risk relatives? Here we can turn to the principles listed earlier. Beneficence and nonmaleficence dictate that one should inform individuals of their risk so as to help them, and to prevent harm. However, informing these relatives without the patient's consent would violate the patient's autonomy, and right to privacy. Furthermore, doing so would also violate the relative's autonomy, as it would deny them their right *not* to know that they are at risk. The issue has been addressed in legal precedent (see Pate v. Thrale, 661 So.2d 278 [Fla.] 1995), which indicate that the physician's obligation is to inform his or her patient of the risk to relatives, but does not necessarily extend the obligation to informing relatives.

Genetic information has been used to discriminate and stigmatize. Long before the discovery of the double helix or Mendel's experiments, people have used genetic information to discriminate and stigmatize groups and individuals. Throughout history, people (usually those with power and/or in the majority) have tried to correlate various traits with genetic inferiority, such as skin color, ethnicity, or cultural identification. Jewish people and people of color (Africans, Asians, Native Americans) have been especially targeted, but individuals with various illnesses (leprosy, AIDS), and physical and developmental handicaps have been the subject of sometimes extreme examples of genetic discrimination, such as the eugenics movement (see below).

Today, genetic discrimination has come to have a different meaning, as worries that genetic test results will be used to limit employment or influence insurance coverage. Although actual occurrences of insurance discrimination are quite rare, this concern is among the most common reasons that people fear genetic testing.

Although these concerns loom large for most people, genetic information is certainly not the only form of medical information that can be used to discriminate against an individual. In fact, HIV status, drug and alcohol history, cholesterol and blood pressure measurements, even height, weight, and age are used by insurers to set rates or even deny coverage, and by employers to hire or fire. Such examples of discrimination illustrate that genetic information is not unique in that it can be used in this manner. Where genetic information is different, however, is that it can be used to discriminate against biologic relatives, be it through the identification of a mutation in a parent or by a pedigree taken during a routine doctor's visit.

Uncovering genetic risk may cause serious psychological harm. Learning that one carries a genetic mutation that predisposes one to cancer, or having a child with mental retardation. may understandably cause anxiety, depression, and fear. For this reason, protocols for some types of genetic testing incorporate psychological counseling as a component. However, it should be obvious that other medical tests, ranging from a biopsy for suspected cancer to an angiogram for coronary artery blockage, can provoke similar emotions.

Although genetic testing provides a very powerful tool for better health, it raises many ethical concerns. These are not novel, but rather can be found in other forms of medical testing. This fact does not make these issues less important, but does serve to emphasize the need for the same strict protection of genetic information as we have for other medical tests. Many argue that the concept of genetic exceptionalism is, in fact, harmful. It gives genetic information a magical aura that, based on the discussion above, it may not deserve. This, in turn, generates both fear and unreasonable expectations among the general public. People may then be reluctant to have genetic testing due to unfounded concerns and, as a consequence, not gain from the benefits that this testing has to offer. For this reason, genetic counseling is a fundamental part of the testing process, so that concerns and expectations are discussed.

GENETIC TESTING OF CHILDREN

Genetic testing for children introduces several ethical issues that are not present when adults undergo genetic testing. Here we are not referring to diagnostic tests, such as the case with VCFS. We are now focusing on predictive genetic testing, which is testing unaffected individuals for later onset disease, such as cancer, or reproductive risks, such as having a child with a birth defect. Adults have the right to know if they carry a genetic mutation that confers for them a high risk for these problems. They are able to make an informed decision that they wish to know this information, based on their assessment of the potential risks (psychological distress, risks for stigmatization, and insurance and employment discrimination) and benefits (for a positive test: earlier and more aggressive screening, medications, prophylactic surgery to reduce or prevent mortality and morbidity, informed family and personal life planning; for a negative test: reduced anxiety, avoid unnecessary screening). Children, however, represent a different situation. Children are not able to make informed decisions on the risks and benefits of this information, so it is the parents who will be making this request, and in doing so they will be violating one important ethical principle, their child's autonomy to decide whether or not to have the genetic testing and learn his or her genetic status at a time when he or she is old enough to make his or her own decision. Is there justification to do that? Does the benefit of learning this information outweigh bypassing the child's right? In most instances bioethicists and genetic professionals believe the answer is "no," and that genetic testing of children for later onset diseases should not be done. For the majority of later onset diseases, there is no medical benefit to learning that a child carries a genetic mutation; there are no recommended screening or treatment protocols that should be initiated in childhood that will limit the occurrence or severity of the disease. However, there are serious potential risks to learning that a child carries this genetic mutation. In addition to the risks described above, a positive test can have significant impact on the child's self-image, parent-child interactions, and the parents or their own expectations regarding education, employment, and personal relations. These are summarized in Table 7-3.

It is assumed that parents will make decisions based on the best interests of their child, and there are many reasons that parents would want their child to have genetic testing for a late onset condition. They may perceive that not doing the testing is in some way keeping a secret from the child, and that it is best for them to tell their child that he or she has this genetic predisposition to a disease. Another argument is that the sooner the child learns of this risk (or eliminates it with a negative test), the easier it will be to move on with his or her life and make appropriate plans. These reasons are grounded in the parent's wish to do the best for their child, but other reasons may be present as well. The parents may want testing in the hope of a negative result to alleviate their guilt of passing the mutation to their child, or to use the information in family planning decisions. In most cases, through genetic counseling, these issues can be explored, identified, and explained so that parents understand the reasons genetic testing for children is not recommended for such diseases.

Therefore, in the absence of a clear medical benefit, genetic testing of children for later onset conditions is not endorsed by the various genetic societies (see Recommended Reading). Similarly, testing children for carrier identification also is not routinely done. Such testing is important only to delineate that child's reproductive risks, and such decisions should be made by that individual when he or she is of an age at which they are able to make an informed decision. This is generally considered during later adolescence, approximately age 16, although this age may vary greatly depending on the maturity of a given individual. Although not of a legal age to consent independently of their parents in many regards, individuals at this age are able to make truly informed decisions and understand the test results at a level at which most genetics health care providers will find it reasonable to perform carrier of later onset disease testing.

GENETIC SCREENING AND EUGENICS

Today, in an effort to reduce or even eradicate certain diseases, we have many genetic screening programs. At their most efficient, they target genetic disorders that are known to occur more commonly in certain ethnic groups, such as Tay-Sachs disease in Ashkenazi Jews or sickle cell disease among African Americans (see Chapter 3). In general these programs are viewed favorably, as they are recognized as trying to eliminate or lessen severe, even fatal, disorders. However, similar sentiments were used once to justify programs that we think of today as morally reprehensible. Based on the concept of eugenics, these programs were intended to better the quality of the human race through selective breeding, selecting for favorable traits, and eliminating unfavorable ones from the gene pool. As farmers and cattleman had done for ages, social scientists in the latter part of the 19th century and early 20th proposed programs to improve the human race. These included the involuntary sterilization of undesirable members of society, such as these labeled "feeble-minded" or criminal. Although it is hard to imagine today, these eugenic programs were widely accepted in the early 20th century. These beliefs were finally discredited with the revelation that eugenics was used to support the Nazi atrocities of World War II.

Although the atrocities done in the name of eugenics are in the past, there are concerns that today we are chasing the same goals. Advances in prenatal genetic diagnosis and assisted reproduction technology has permitted what some argue are "designer babies." These technologies have allowed many couples at risk for having children with severe genetic disease to have healthy children. However, companies now market the ability to select a baby's sex, and many are concerned that other nondisease traits will soon follow, such as intelligence or physical attractiveness. Although the reality is that we have a very limited understanding of these very complex traits, the prospect that one day we may be able to select many traits for a child is not inconceivable. It should be evident then that debates on the ethical issues will certainly continue, hopefully in advance of the progress in genetic technology.

RECOMMENDED READING

Clayton, E. (2003). Ethical, legal, and social implications of genomic medicine. *New England Journal of Medicine, 349*(6), 562–569.

Falk, M. J., Dugan, R. B., O'Riorday, M. A., & Robin, N. H. (2003). Medical geneticists' duty to warn at-risk relatives for genetic disease. *American Journal of Medical Genetics, 120*A(3), 374–380.

Green, M. J., & Botkin, J. R. (2003). "Genetic exceptionalism" in medicine: Clarifying the differences between genetic and non genetic tests. *Annals of Internal Medicine, 138*(7), 571–575.

Martin, R. (2001). How distinctive is genetic information? *Studies in History and Philosophy of Biological and Biomedical Science, 32*, 663-687.

Murray, T. H. (1997). Genetic exceptionalism and future diaries: Is genetic information different from other medical information? In M. A. Rothstein (Ed.), *Genetic secrets: Protecting privacy and confidentiality in the genetic era* (pp. 60-73). New Haven, CT: Yale University Press.

Pellegrin, E. D. (1999). Clinicat éthiques consultations. *Journal of Clinical Ethics, 10*, 5-13.

Pence, G. H. (2004). *Classical cases in medical ethics* (4th ed.). Boston: McGraw-Hill.

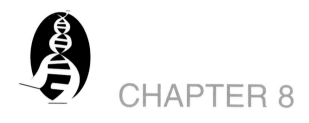

CHAPTER 8

Genetic Counseling and Your Practice

NATHANIEL H. ROBIN, MD
SANDRA PRUCKA, CGC

Genetic counseling is the process of helping people understand and adapt to the medical, psychological and familial implications of genetic contributions to disease. This process integrates:

■ *Interpretation of family and medical histories to assess the chance of disease occurrence or recurrence.*

■ *Education about inheritance, testing, management, prevention, resources and research.*

■ *Counseling to promote informed choices and adaptation to the risk or condition.*

National Society of Genetic Counselors (2005)

HISTORY AND ORGANIZATION OF GENETIC COUNSELING

Although the profession of genetic counseling is relatively young, genetic counseling as a concept emerged in the post-World War II era. The term "genetic counseling" was first introduced in 1947, almost a decade prior to the identification of the correct chromosome number as 46 in 1956. At that time, the science of genetics was viewed negatively, owing to its association with the eugenics movement and the atrocities carried out by scientists in Nazi Germany. Concern remained that genetics would be used to discriminate and even eliminate those who were considered "genetically inferior."

The underlying principles of modern genetic counseling were developed in response to these fears, and genetic counseling emerged as a profession. Genetic counselors are driven by a nondirective approach to genetic counseling, which emphasizes patient autonomy in decision making (see Chapter 7, Ethical Issues in Genetic Testing). This not only allows but encourages a patient to make the personal decision regarding his or her health care, especially regarding genetic testing, after a thorough discussion of the benefits, risks, limitations, and implications involved.

For years many individuals from a variety of backgrounds provided genetic counseling to patients. Today, however, genetic counseling is a recognized separate masters-level health care specialty. The first program began at Sarah Lawrence College in 1969, and there are now 27 masters-level genetic counseling programs in the United States, as well as programs in the United Kingdom, Canada, and Australia. The number of programs has continued to grow over the years and this growth is anticipated to continue into the future. The American Board of Genetic Counseling (ABGC) has been the overall credentialing body for the genetic counseling profession since 1993. Credentialing for the profession includes accrediting new programs to ensure they meet the standards of training for the profession, recertification of existing programs, as well as certification and recertification of genetic counselors after their graduation from an accredited program. Through credentialing, the ABGC is able to ensure there is a standard competence for clinical practice for genetic counselors, which not only benefits the public but also advances the profession.

In addition to the ABGC, there is a national organization that serves as the professional membership association for the genetic counseling profession. This organization is called the National Society of Genetic Counselors (NSGC) and was created in 1979. The NSGC serves as a voice for genetic counselors through professional advocacy and leadership with their overall mission being to "promote the genetic counseling profession as a recognized and integral part of health care delivery, education, research and public policy" (http://www.nsgc.org).

AREAS OF PRACTICE FOR GENETIC COUNSELORS

Due to the increasing importance of genetics in the evaluation of their patients, it is important for audiologists, speech-language pathologists, and otolaryngologists to have an understanding and appreciation for the role that genetic counselors play in patient care. Genetic counselors are not limited to patient care. Many are active in other activities, such as research, laboratory, government, administrative, and teaching roles. However, it is through patient care that they will most likely interact with audiologists, speech-language pathologists, and otolaryngologists, so we focus on the clinical roles of genetic counselors.

Genetic counselors work in various clinical settings that include preconception, prenatal, pediatric, adult, and metabolic genetic counseling. Each of these categories is general and could be further subdivided into myriad specialty clinics in which medical genetics is active, such as skeletal dysplasias, cleft and craniofacial disorders, and hereditary cancer clinics (see Chapter 2). Although a genetic counselors role in each clinic may differ, the profession as a whole is governed by several underlying principles. Among these is an emphasis on proper pre- and post-test genetic counseling. It is through this process that patients are fully informed before and after going forward with genetic counseling, ensuring that they can make an independent and informed decision (Table 8-1). As part of this process, genetic counselors ensure that patients have access to resources for additional information and support.

THE UNDERLYING PRINCIPLES OF GENETIC COUNSELING: NONDIRECTIVE GENETIC COUNSELING

Genetic counselors believe that all patients have the right to make their own decision regarding genetic evaluation and genetic testing without outside influence or persuasion from biased sources, such as that provided by other family members, the health care providers, financial concerns, and even societal pressures. Although on a practical level it is impossible to isolate a patient entirely from all of these external factors, genetic counselors strive to provide

TABLE 8–1. The Process of Pre- and Post-Test Genetic Counseling

Pretest genetic counseling	The process of proving detailed information regarding the risks, benefits, and limitations of pursuing genetic testing in a supportive environment. The patient and his or her family are given information regarding appropriate testing options and are provided guidance through the testing process.
Post-test genetic counseling	Supportive counseling provided to a patient and their family after pursuing genetic counseling. The genetic counselor reviews the interpretation of the test result and its relevance to the patient as well as his or her immediate and extended family members. In the event of a positive result, clinical relevance is discussed as well as appropriate management and resources for support. In the event of a negative result, the genetic counselor, and often physician as well, will discuss any additional testing options and implications of a negative result. Careful attention is paid to the psychosocial impact either result has for the child and the family unit.

unbiased and accurate information to patients. The goal of genetic counseling is to facilitate informed decision making. It is through this process that patients are provided with a comprehensive understanding of the testing options that are appropriate for them. This discussion includes basic science information (i.e., definition of chromosomes, genes, inheritance patterns, etc.) as well as a discussion of the risks, benefits, and limitations of testing. This approach is intended to allow patients to make a decision regarding whether or not to pursue testing that is best for their personal and family situation. It is important that the genetic counselor discloses all relevant information throughout this process and is not selective in what information is provided during the counseling session. The term used to describe this process is "nondirective" genetic counseling. This approach works to provide guidance as to the appropriateness of genetic testing, and is clearly distinct from the dated paternalistic medical model in which the healthcare provider makes the decision as to what plan of medical management is best for a patient.

In addition to informing patients about genetic testing, genetic counselors work to provide access to genetic services. Genetic testing is not always covered by insurance providers and it can be especially difficult for those with Medicare, Medicaid, or no insurance. Genetic counselors often work with patients to investigate their coverage, and advocate for them with insurance companies, explaining why these tests are indeed necessary for optimum medical management.

GENETIC COUNSELING FOR PEDIATRIC DEAFNESS

Pretest Genetic Counseling

There are several key components to the pretest counseling of patients with pediatric deafness (Table 8-2). As with all genetic counseling sessions, it is first important to assess the family's understanding of why they have been referred for genetic counseling. This allows the counselor to understand what prior information the family may be coming to the session with and helps the counselor begin to elucidate the main concerns the family has regarding their child's diagnosis. During this time with the family, medical and family history information is gathered and some initial information regarding the causes of pediatric deafness is discussed.

The pretest genetic counseling session also allows the counselor time to assess the family's cultural beliefs, cultural hearing status, ethnicity, socioeconomic status, and other factors that may influence the family's approach to healthcare. Regardless of the context of the genetic counseling session, genetic counselors are sensitive to how these factors may influence the needs of their patients. Within the context of counseling for pediatric hearing, it is especially important to assess if a deaf/hard-of-hearing family identifies with

TABLE 8–2. Components of Pretest Genetic Counseling for Pediatric Deafness

---

Assess family's understanding of the reason for referral to genetics

Obtain a copy of the patient's audiograms

Obtain an accurate family and medical history

- Special attention is paid to elucidating information regarding symptoms that can be seen with syndromic forms of hearing loss (i.e. early onset arthritis seen with Stickler syndrome or renal anomalies that may suggest Alport syndrome or Branchiootorenal syndrome)

Discuss causes of deafness with the family

- Review definition of chromosomes and genes
- Explain the different genetic and non-genetic causes of deafness
- Discuss the difference between syndromic and non-syndromic

Physical examination is performed by the geneticist

Recommendations for testing are discussed with the family

- Informed consent is obtained prior to proceeding with genetic testing (risks, benefits and limitations of testing are discussed)

---

the cultural deaf community, referred to as Deaf (upper case letter "D," Deaf community, or Deaf culture). This is especially important because 5 to 10% of deaf children have one or both deaf parents, and have a higher likelihood of identifying with the Deaf community/culture. Individuals who consider themselves Deaf do not look at deafness as a disability but have a positive view toward their deafness and share a common sense of pride in their culture, sharing a common language, values, and identity (see Deaf Culture). It is, therefore, important as a genetic counselor or other medical professional working with individuals who are hard-of-hearing, deaf, or Deaf to communicate with the patient and his or her family prior to their appointment to determine their preferred language of communication and, if requested, to arrange for an interpreter who is educated in sign language (American Sign Language or British Sign Language). It is important that a family member is not used to facilitate this communication process, as they may harbor certain biases that do not allow for an accurate communication of information between the counselor and the family.

In addition to considering the communication needs of their clients, genetic counselors work to understand the cultural communities they work with and pay particular attention to omitting words, mannerisms, and practices that may be offensive to these groups. For example, when working with the deaf community, it is important to refer to individuals as being deaf or hard-of-hearing, instead of using words such as "affected" and "unaffected," as well as to pay particular attention to avoiding words such as "impairment" or

---

The Deaf Culture

Individuals who identify with this cultural community refer to themselves as Deaf individuals, where the uppercase letter "D" is used to signify that this is a distinct cultural community. Members of the Deaf community share a common language, called American Sigh Language (although there are closely related sign languages in non-English-speaking countries), as well as common cultural values and beliefs. Deaf individuals view deafness as part of their identity and share a common sense of pride in being deaf, and this creates an environment where deaf individuals can feel understood and accepted. The concepts of shared language, Deaf pride, and Deaf identity form the foundation of the Deaf culture.

"pathology." These words imply that deafness is an impairment or condition, whereas members of the Deaf community do not view deafness in this manner, and it is important to respect their cultural beliefs.

Parental Knowledge and Concern

Parents often discuss what they feel has contributed to their child's hearing loss during the pretest genetic counseling session. Although "parents" in this section refers to hearing parents who have a child with deafness, there are also concerns surrounding deaf parents having children with and without deafness, and this will be explored in other areas of this chapter.

It is not uncommon for parents to express concern that they somehow caused their child's deafness due to something they did or did not do during the pregnancy. In addition, parents often are also concerned about whether or not their child's hearing loss will progress, whether or not it will be associated with other health concerns or with intellectual impairment, and what their risks are for future pregnancies. Genetic testing can address these concerns and often can provide some reassurance to the family. A study by Brunger et al. in 2000 found that 96% of the 96 individuals surveyed expressed a positive attitude toward genetic testing with 76% stating that they were interested in having genetic testing themselves. The most common reason given for their interest in pursuing genetic testing in this study was to identify the cause of their child's hearing loss, while the second and third most common reasons were to refine their recurrence risks for future pregnancies and better understand their child's future medical management and/or treatment. Although genetic testing can help to answer some of these parental concerns, it is important that this information accompany appropriate pre-

and post-test genetic counseling to avoid misinterpretation of this information. For example, in the same study by Brunger et al., it was shown that as many as 32% of individuals who had received genetic testing incorrectly interpreted the information they were given. Some misinterpreted the meaning of a negative genetic test; others inaccurately estimated the recurrence risks for themselves, their affected children, and extended family members. The pretest counseling session is an essential time for the genetic counselor to explain the potential outcomes of genetic testing and the implication of these results to the patient and his or her family members. The counselor uses a variety of techniques during these sessions so that information is both communicated to, and understood by, the patient and family. For example, techniques such as rephrasing, reflecting, and promoting shared language are interviewing techniques that enhance the family's comfort and trust of the counselor and allow for a focused and informative counseling session for all parties involved in this communication process.

PARENTAL INTEREST IN GENETIC TESTING FOR DEAFNESS

A number of studies have examined the interest of individuals in genetic testing, both to better define the etiology of their (or their child's) hearing loss/deafness and to use this information for prenatal testing. In this section, we describe parents' interest in pursuing genetic testing to better define the etiology of their child's hearing loss from the perspective of hearing parents and of those who are themselves hard-of-hearing/deaf/Deaf.

Hard-of-Hearing, deaf, and Deaf Parents

There are differing views of deafness in the medical community and the Deaf community. The traditional medical model views deafness as a condition that needs to be treated or cured. Those who identify as part of the Deaf community, however, feel that deafness should be preserved and understood from a cultural perspective. Individuals who are part of the Deaf community/culture have, therefore, been distrustful of the field of genetics due to the fear that genetic testing will lead to a depletion of individuals in their community. This was illustrated in a study conducted by Middleton, Hewison, and Mueller. (1998), which examined the attitudes of deaf adults toward genetic testing for hereditary deafness by interviewing a group of well-educated people attending the "Deaf Nation" conference at the University of Central Lancashire in 1997, where the emphasis of this conference was on Deaf cultural issues. The majority of the 87 individuals surveyed had an overall negative view toward genetic testing, with their main concerns being that genetic testing would do more harm than good and would devalue deaf individuals. This study also found that those with deafness who did not consider themselves culturally Deaf (these individuals do not exclusively associate with the Deaf community and are referred to in this section as "deaf") also had a negative view toward genetic testing, but were more likely to be neutral toward this issue. A number of studies published since the Middleton study also have examined the opinions of deaf and Deaf individuals toward genetic testing (Guillemin & Gillam, 2006; Stern et al., 2002; Taneja, Padya, Foley, Nicely, & Arnos, 2004). These studies found that both groups seem to have demonstrated a more positive, or at least neutral, view toward genetic testing than originally reported in the Middleton et al. study. These studies do point out, however, that individuals who identify most with the Deaf community are more likely than deaf individuals to feel that genetic testing will have an overall negative effect on the deaf community.

Regardless of their views toward genetic testing, recent studies have shown that individuals from both groups stress the importance of fully informing those pursuing genetic testing of all the aspects of deafness prior to going forward. In one study (Guillemin & Gillam, 2006), individuals explained that this educational session with families should include not only information on the experiences of deaf individuals but also medical and technologic options for deaf individuals as well as options for communication and education. They emphasized that this open discussion with families should allow them to make an informed personal choice regarding genetic testing given this comprehensive view of deafness. Although genetic counselors alone are not trained to provide all the technologic options for hearing-impaired individuals, it is this type of informed decision making that is the cornerstone of genetic counseling. Both the pre- and post-test genetic counseling sessions allow for this type of in-depth discussion with families to ensure a comprehensive view throughout the testing process. It is through this process that counselors are also able to refer families to meet with experts who work with deaf individuals as well as to provide contact information for families to meet with individuals who are deaf/hard-of-hearing/Deaf to ensure that all their questions are answered prior to undergoing genetic testing.

Although there appears to be an overall positive or neutral view toward genetic testing for deafness in both deaf and Deaf groups, there is understandable caution especially from the Deaf community that genetic testing for deafness could ultimately lead to fewer children with deafness, thereby depleting their community. A genetic counselor working with deaf and Deaf individuals must consider these viewpoints and be sensitive to these views when working with deaf/Deaf individuals and their families.

Hearing Parents

A number of studies also have looked at the opinions of hearing parents of children who are hard-of-hearing/deaf toward genetic testing for hearing loss (Brunger et al., 2000; Burton, Withrow, Amos, Kalfoglu, & Pandya, 2006;

Dagan, O'Hochner, Levi, Raas-Rothchild, & Sagi, 2002; Parker, Fortnam, Young, & Davis., 2000). Most of these studies, including Brunger et al. (2000), found that the majority of those surveyed have a positive view toward genetic testing. Some of these studies have demonstrated that individuals are interested in pursuing genetic testing for their children to help them better understand the etiology of their child's hearing loss, aid in determining if there is a risk for other family members to have deafness, and aid in research to promote treatment of hearing loss/deafness.

In general, these attitudes toward genetic testing are in sharp contrast with those observed in the Deaf community. However, although the majority of hearing parents have a positive view toward genetic testing, some do share common concerns with individuals of the hard-of-hearing, deaf, and Deaf communities. These concerns center on the perception that genetic testing is a first step toward prenatal diagnosis and pregnancy termination due to hearing status. The interesting issue of prenatal diagnosis for hearing loss will be discussed in greater detail in the next section.

Post-Test Genetic Counseling

During the post-test genetic counseling session, the genetic counselor discusses the relevance of the patient's test results with the patient and/or his or her family members (in the case of minors). This can be done in one of several ways, depending on the institution's policy regarding the method of disclosing these results to patients. In some instances, a follow-up appointment to discuss these results is scheduled at the end of the patient's pretest counseling session. In other instances, the patient/family is called with these results and then asked to come in to discuss the test results in greater detail during a follow-up appointment. Regardless of the method used to communicate these test results to the patient, this plan is established and discussed with the patient during the pretest counseling session. As with the pretest genetic counseling session, there are several key components to the post-test counseling session, which are outlined in Table 8–3.

Impact of Results on Parents and Families

The post-test genetic counseling session is an important time to reemphasize concepts covered during the pretest session and relate them to the patient's specific test results and personal situation. If the test results are positive, it gives the counselor and physician time to review the meaning of a positive result. Concepts such as recurrence risk, medical management, and overall outcome are discussed with the family. In addition, now that the genetic cause of deafness in the family has been identified, this result can be used to test other family members. The genetic counselor plays an essential role in explaining inheritance patterns, identifying individuals who would benefit

TABLE 8–3. Components of Post-Test Genetic Counseling for Pediatric Deafness

Discussion of a positive test result
- Discuss associated medical aspects (i.e., progressive vs. nonprogressive, associated health complications, etc.)
- Discuss impact on medical management
- Recurrence risk counseling
- Discuss inheritance and at-risk family members
- Prenatal testing options for future pregnancies

Discussion of a negative test result
- Emphasize that a negative test result does not mean that their child's deafness is not genetic
- Discuss additional testing options and the need for continued follow-up with
- genetics recurrence risk counseling

Seek feedback from the family regardless of testing outcome
- Impact of test result for the patient's family
- Verify that information was not rejected based on prior beliefs

Refer the family to local and national support groups

from genetic counseling to discuss their testing options, and facilitating genetic counseling/testing for interested family members locally, or in their state or country of origin. A positive test result also means that prenatal genetic testing becomes an option for the parents and other at-risk and interested family members. Genetic counselors assist in explaining these options to couples and facilitating prenatal testing as well.

If the test results are negative, it is important for the family to understand that there still may be a hereditary cause for their child/family member's deafness and, if clinically relevant, additional testing options to investigate this risk are often discussed during the post-test counseling session. In addition, although it is often difficult to provide recurrence risk information with a negative result, empiric risk data may be available, which can be communicated to the family during this post-test counseling session (see Chapter 9).

Regardless of test outcome, the post-test session allows time for the counselor to assess the impact that the test results, and the testing process as a whole, has had for the patient and his or her family. It is often difficult for the family to reject past beliefs of what may have caused their child's deafness to accept a positive test result. Therefore, the post-test session is an essential time for the genetic counselor to verify that the information gained from the testing process is not rejected by the family based on these prior beliefs. Just as with the pretest session, genetic counselors use specific counseling techniques to promote this communication process and to be certain that the family understands the implications of the test result. The uniqueness of genetic testing is that this result has implications for the immediate and extended family, not just the individual undergoing testing. Therefore, the counselor often assists with communicating this information to other family members and/or locating resources for counseling and support in their area.

PRENATAL TESTING

As discussed above, parents often come to a genetic counseling session with questions concerning risks to future offspring. If a genetic cause for deafness has been identified, prenatal testing often can provide answers to these questions without parents having to wait for newborn hearing screening.

Prenatal testing for hearing status is a sensitive issue in both the hearing, hard-of-hearing/deaf, and Deaf communities. One role of the genetic coun-

---

Deaf Parents Seeking a Child with Deafness

In 2002, there was an article that featured a lesbian couple searching for a deaf sperm donor in the hope that this selection process would increase their changes of having a child, who, like themselves, was deaf. This article appeared in the *Washington Post Magazine* and created a firestorm of ethical debates regarding the use of genetic testing by individuals with deafness, or other conditions with a hereditary component, to have children who are similarly affected. Consider the following scenario:

> A deaf couple comes in for genetic counseling to learn the etiology of their hearing loss. They explain to the genetic counselor that they are interested in determining the cause of their deafness so that they can pursue prenatal testing that will select for a child who is deaf.

■ Would you feel differently about this scenario if it was a hearing couple seeking genetic counseling to select against having a child with deafness?

■ Should this couple have the same right to have a child with a similar background as a couple seeking prenatal testing to select against a child with Down syndrome? Spina bifida? A lethal genetic condition?

■ Would you consider this decision abusive or selfishly disabling?

selor is to inform families of their risks for a genetically determined trait to be transmitted to future generations. As such, the issue of prenatal testing is an integral part of the post-test counseling session and often spills over to additional sessions with a prenatal genetic counselor to explore the option of prenatal testing in greater detail. Through an examination of the literature, or in conversations with individuals from the different communities discussed above, strikingly different opinions and beliefs become apparent regarding prenatal testing for hearing status. Some individuals in the deaf/hard-of-hearing, and Deaf communities would consider prenatal testing in an effort to conceive a child with deafness just as some individuals who are hearing parents may be interested in prenatal testing to conceive a child who is also hearing (see Deaf Parents Seeking a Child with Deafness). There are also members of each of these communities who believe genetic testing for hearing status should only be used postnatally. Genetic counselors are aware of these opposing viewpoints and specially equipped to sensitively explore these topics with patients and their family members.

GENETIC TESTING OF MINORS

As described throughout this section, the genetic counselor plays an integral role in identifying at-risk family members who would benefit from genetic counseling and testing during the post-testing counseling session. During this counseling process, it is not uncommon for a parent to ask if an unaffected minor could be tested to determine his or her risks of having future children with the genetic condition that has been identified in the family. There are many reasons that this occurs. Parents may be concerned about their child's risks for future pregnancies, they may want this information to enhance their ability to communicate and relate information regarding the genetic condition in the family to their child, or they may want this time for their child to adjust to the information of being a carrier of a genetic condition. Keeping these views in mind, it is also important to consider the child's needs and the risks and benefits of carrier testing.

The American Society of Human Genetics, American College of Medical Genetics, and National Society of Genetic Counselors all have guidelines regarding this issue and hold the common belief that genetic testing should only be performed on minors when a medical or psychosocial benefit to the child can be demonstrated. Issues such as a child's self-perceptions, peer identification, loss of confidentiality, and autonomous decision making are clear psychosocial issues that the genetic counselor considers before determining the benefit of carrier testing for minors. Genetic counselors are specially trained in facilitating an open communication process that both enables the family to express their concerns as well as to understand the complexities of testing minors and the psychosocial harm that can result.

The advent of prenatal testing for genetic conditions such as cystic fibrosis, sickle cell disease, and even hearing loss now makes it possible for incidental carrier status to be identified. Parents seeking prenatal genetic testing may learn that the fetus is a carrier of a mutation for an autosomal recessive genetic condition. This poses an interesting dilemma, as it is an ethically complex question if this information should be disclosed to the child. Genetic counselors work with families in this situation to determine the appropriate time to disclose this information for each family, and often assist in disclosing the information within the context of a genetic counseling session so that the family can ensure that up-to-date accurate information is disclosed at the time this conversation takes place.

SUPPORT

Both the pre- and post-test genetic counseling sessions are ideal times for the genetic counselor to provide support to the family and identify resources for additional support on the community, state, and national levels. Support can mean anything from referring patients for personal and/or family therapy to connecting with groups of individuals affected with a common genetic condition. In the case of deafness, genetic counselors assist in identifying community groups of those who are also deaf/hard-of-hearing/Deaf, assist in identifying medical professionals who can help assess their child's deafness and provide continued care, and connect parents with other individuals and/or families affected by deafness. Genetic counselors are, therefore, great community resources for families as well as for other medical professionals.

REFERENCES

Brunger J. W., Murray, G. S., O'Riordan, M., Mathews, A. L,, Smith, R. J. H., & Robin, N. H. (2000). Parental attitudes toward genetic testing for pediatric deafness. *American Journal of Human Genetics*, *67*, 1621–1625.

Burton, S. K., Withrow, K., Arnos, K. S., Kalfoglou, A. L., & Pandya, A. (2006). A focus group study of consumer attitudes toward genetic testing and newborn screening for deafness. *Genetics in Medicine*, *8*(12), 779–783.

Dagan, O., Hochner, H., Levi, H., Raas-Rothschild, A., & Sagi, M. (2002). Genetic testing for hearing loss: Different motivations for the same outcome. *American Journal of Medical Genetics*, *113*, 137–143.

Guillemin, M., & Gillam, L. (2006). Attitudes to genetic testing for deafness: The importance of informed choice. *Journal of Genetic Counseling*, *15*(1), 51–59.

Middleton, A., Hewison, J., & Mueller, R. F. (1998). Attitudes of deaf adults toward genetic testing for hereditary deafness. *American Journal of Human Genetics*, *63*, 1175–1180.

Parker, M. J., Fortnum, H. M., Young, I. D., & Davis, A. C. (2000). Genetics and deafness: What do families want? *Journal of Medical Genetics, 37*, E26.

Stern, S. J., Arno, S. K., Murrelle, L., Oelrich Welch, K., Nance, W. E., & Pandya, A. (2002). Attitudes of deaf and hard of hearing subjects towards genetic testing and prenatal diagnosis of hearing loss. *Journal of Medical Genetics, 39*, 449–453.

Taneja, P. R., Padya, A., Foley, D. L., Nicely, L. V., & Arnos, K. S. (2004). Attitudes of deaf individuals towards genetic testing. *American Journal of Medical Genetics, 130A*, 17–21.

RECOMMENDED READING

ACMG statement by the Genetic Evaluation of Congenital Hearing Loss Expert Panel. (2002). Genetics evaluation guidelines for the etiologic diagnosis of congenital hearing loss. *Genetics in Medicine, 4*(3), 162–171.

American Board of Genetic Counseling. http://www.abgc.net

Baker, D. L., Schuette, J. L., & Uhlmann, W. R. (1998). *A guide to genetic counseling.* New York: John Wiley and Sons.

Bauman, H. D. (2005). Designing deaf babies and the question of disability. *Journal of Deaf Studies and Deaf Education, 10*(3), 311–315.

Chapple, A., May, C., & Campion, P. (1995). Lay understanding of genetic disease: A British study of families attending a genetic counseling service. *Journal of Genetic Counseling, 4*(4), 281–300.

Heimler, A. (1997). An oral history of the National Society of Genetic Counselors. *Journal of Genetic Counseling, 6*(3), 315–336.

Joint Committee on Infant Hearing. (2000). Year 2000 position statement: Principles and guidelines for early hearing detection and intervention programs. *Pediatrics, 106*, 798–817.

McConkie-Rosell, A., & Spiridigliozzi, G. A. (2004). Family matters: A conceptual framework for genetic testing in children. *Journal of Genetic Counseling, 13*(1), 9–29.

McCreary Stebnicki, J. A., & Coeling, H. V. (1999). The culture of the Deaf. *Journal of Transcultural Nursing, 10*(4), 350–357.

Middleton, A, Hewison, J., & Mueller, R. (2001). Prenatal diagnosis for inherited deafness—What is the potential demand? *Journal of Genetic Counseling, 10*(2), 121–131.

National Society of Genetic Counselors. (2005). http://www.nsgc.org

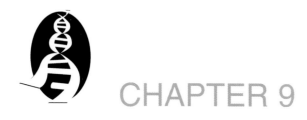

CHAPTER 9

Genetics and Hearing Loss

*T*he final three chapters of this book each discuss focused topics. This chapter provides a review of the genetic evaluation of the child with sensorineural hearing impairment. Chapter 10 focuses on cleft lip and cleft palate, and Chapter 11 on more extensive craniofacial anomalies, such as craniosynostosis. Although covering distinct material, each chapter has several common themes. First is how a geneticist differentiates syndromic from nonsyndromic. Then, after that determination is made, what are the important genetic issues for each scenario—what testing is recommended, and what counseling can be offered.

INTRODUCTION

Hearing impairment is both a common and complex disorder, requiring a multidisciplinary team approach to provide affected individuals the best opportunity for favorable speech and language development. Although the respective roles of the otolaryngologist, audiologist, and speech-language pathologist are obvious, the role of the geneticist is less clear. Until recently, this discussion would have been very brief, focused entirely on genetic syndromes that are associated with hearing impairment. However, the geneticist's role has greatly expanded. In the last decade, tremendous advances have been made in our understanding of the genetic basis of sensorineural hearing impairment. With these genetic discoveries has come a greater understanding of disorders of hearing, and with that many new genetically based tests for many different forms of hearing impairment. For this reason a genetic evaluation has become an integral part of the initial evaluation of all hearing-impaired individuals. Even for those who have isolated hearing impairment, this evaluation can provide very useful information.

AN OVERVIEW OF HEARING IMPAIRMENT

It is not the intent of this chapter to provide a comprehensive review of hearing impairment. We do not provide a review of the normal anatomy and physiology of the hearing process nor discuss in detail the various techniques of audiologic evaluation. We assume that the reader has a general understanding of these areas. Furthermore, there are many excellent reviews that discuss these topics in detail, several of which are listed at the end of this chapter. Rather, what follows is a brief overview that is intended to provide the background necessary to understand what follows regarding the genetic basis of hearing.

EPIDEMIOLOGY

Sensorineural hearing impairment is the most commonly reported sensory deficit. In the United States, approximately 1 in 1000 infants are born with significant hearing impairment. The impact of hearing impairment for the child, his or her family, and the health care system cannot be overstated. The lifetime costs for a child born with a significant hearing impairment exceeds $1 million. Furthermore, even mild degrees of hearing impairment have been shown to have an adverse effect on the individual's educational outcome, future employment, future earnings, use of the health care system, and even life expectancy.

Early and accurate identification has been shown to be a necessary component for favorable speech and language development. A diagnosis made after 6 months of age has an adverse long-term impact on speech and language potential. This fact has been one of the driving forces for universal newborn screening for hearing impairment.

TERMINOLOGY

Many terms are used interchangeably when discussing disorders of hearing. Here, we use the term "hearing impairment" to mean any deficit in one's ability to hear, whereas "hearing loss" implies that an individual had normal hearing, but lost some or all of that ability; "deaf" implies an individual has no hearing; "hard of hearing" refers to any level of hearing impairment. Some groups, notably the Deaf (upper case "D") community,[1] express concern that

---

[1]The Deaf community is a vibrant cultural group whose long-standing traditions and customs are based on their use of sign language to communicate. Most members were born deaf, often to deaf parents. To the Deaf, the lack of hearing is a normal state, central to their culture, not as a medical disease. They view negatively anything that suggests that lack of hearing is a medical disease, including efforts to treat or cure it.

terms such as "hearing impairment" have a negative connotation. It is certainly not our intention in using this term to be insensitive to the Deaf community, or any other group. Rather, we use it for clarity in indicating what type of hearing problem is being discussed.

CLASSIFICATION

Once the diagnosis of hearing impairment is confirmed by formal audiologic testing, the exact type of hearing impairment should be further classified by several parameters. These are listed in Table 9-1, and include severity and frequency, anatomical location, age of onset, and etiology.

The severity and frequency of the hearing impairment is determined in the course of the audiologic testing, and reflects the threshold and frequency range at which the individual can perceive sound. The severity of the hearing impairment is classified by the intensity level of the sound (in decibels, dB) that the individual can detect. Results are graded as mild (20-40 dB), moderate (41-55 dB), moderately severe (56-70 dB), severe (71-90 dB), and profound (>90 dB). Although there is no universally accepted designation, individuals with severe-to-profound hearing impairment are often considered "deaf," while those with lesser degrees of hearing impairment are termed "hard of hearing."

TABLE 9–1. The Parameters of Sensorineural Hearing Impairment

Anatomic and functional location
- Conductive
- Sensorineural
- Mixed (components of both conductive and sensorineural)

Severity
- Mild to moderate (20–40 dB)
- Moderate (41–55 dB)
- Moderately severe (56–70 dB)
- Severe (71–90 dB)
- Profound (>90 dB)

Age of onset
- Before language development/before age 3 years (prelingual, including congenital)
- Later onset / progressive

Syndromic (associated with other anomalies) or isolated

Frequency is a measure of sound pitch, with tests typically running from 250 Hertz (Hz) (a low bass sound) to 8000 Hz (a squeak). Normal speech occurs between 500 to 4000 Hz at approximately 25 to 35 dB. Establishing the degree and frequencies of hearing impairment is important for management planning and determining etiology.

The anatomic location of a hearing deficit often reflects whether the hearing impairment is conductive (a disorder of the external or middle ear), sensorineural (a disorder involving the inner ear and/or central nervous system), or mixed (with elements of both types). Conductive hearing impairment can be caused by middle ear infections but also complete aural atresia, as can be found in Treacher Collins syndrome, a type of syndromic deafness.

It is also important to establish age of onset. Hearing impairment that is detected before the acquisition of speech is classified as prelingual, whereas hearing loss that is diagnosed in individuals after the acquisition of speech is referred to as late-onset. Some types of late-onset hearing loss can be due to genetic factors.

It is also important to try to establish causality. About half of hearing impairment is due to "environmental" factors (Figure 9–1). Examples include congenital cytomegalovirus disease and noise-induced hearing loss. The latter is more accurately described as "multifactorial," as genetic background clearly plays a role in its development.

About half of deafness is genetic. This diagnosis implies that the hearing impairment is caused by a genetic change. When considering genetic hearing impairment, a primary question is to ask if it is associated with other medical

---

Environmental (~50%)
    Congenital infection (CMV, rubella)
    Prematurity
    Ototoxic medications (aminoglycosides)
Genetic (50%)2
    Syndromic (30%)
        Hunter syndrome
        FGFR3-related craniosynostosis (Muenke syndrome)
        Stickler syndrome
        Treacher Collins syndrome
    Nonsyndromic (70%)
        70% - autosomal recessive (symbol: DFNB)
        25% - autosomal dominant (symbol: DFNA)
        1% - X-linked (symbol: DFN)
        1% - Mitochondrial (no symbol)

FIGURE 9–1. Prelingual hearing impairment.

problems. These types of hearing impairment are known as syndromic. If it is not associated with any other medical problems, it is referred to as isolated or nonsyndromic.

SYNDROMIC HEARING IMPAIRMENT

Several hundred genetic syndromes have hearing impairment as one component manifestation, and in aggregate, these syndromes account for about 30% of genetic deafness. An abbreviated list is provided in Table 9–2, and a more complete list may be found in the Hereditary Hearing Loss Home Page (2007). Some syndromes are easily recognized; others are subtle. For this reason, the evaluation of a person with hearing impairment must be careful and systematic. Several of the more common genetic syndromes that present with hearing impairment are discussed.

- **Hunter syndrome** is an X-linked disorder caused by deficiency of the enzyme iduronate-2-sulfatase. This deficiency leads to a toxic accumulation of mucopolysaccharides (MPS) in various organs and tissues of the body, including the brain. Affected boys manifest coarse facial characteristics, enlargement of the liver and spleen, and significant developmental delay (Figure 9–2). Hunter syndrome is only one of several types of MPS disorders, and in all hearing impairment is a common associated manifestation.

- **Muenke syndrome**, also called Adelaide-type craniosynostosis, is an autosomal dominant disorder caused by a specific mutation in the gene fibroblast growth factor receptor 3 (FGFR3). Although many affected persons have an obviously abnormal skull shape due to early closure of the coronal sutures (two of the joints of the skull bones at which head growth occurs in early childhood.) Such children may also have an abnormal facial appearance, and hand and foot anomalies. Interestingly, some people who carry the same mutation have milder physical findings, and some even manifest only hearing impairment. Other mutations in FGFR3 cause a variety of skeletal disorders, such as achondroplasia, and mutations in other FGFR's cause other syndromes that have overlap with Muenke, such as Apert, Crouzon, and Pfeiffer syndromes. These are discussed in more detail in Chapter 11.

- **Cleidocranial dysplasia** is another autosomal dominant syndrome hearing impairment. It is caused by mutations in the *RUNX2* gene. Although the craniofacial appearance may be less dramatic than seen with Muenke or Hunter syndromes, the associated findings

TABLE 9–2. Select Syndromes with Hearing Impairment

- Abruzzo-Erickson
- acroosteolysis
- Achondroplasia
- Adelaide/FGFR3
- Apert
- auralcephalosyndactyly
- auro-digital-anal
- Boston-type craniosynostosis
- branchio-oto-renal
- campomelic dysplasia
- Camurati-Engelmann
- cat eye
- cervico-oculo-acoustic
- CHARGE
- cleidocranial dysplasia
- Cockayne
- cranial sclerosis
- craniodiaphyseal dys
- craniometaphyseal dys
- Crouzon
- del(18q)
- EEC
- facio-auriculo-radial dys
- focal dermal hypoplasia
- Fountain
- frontometaphyseal dys
- glactosialidosis
- gengival fibromatosis
- Hersh
- hyperphosphatasemia
- hypertelorism-microtia-clefting
- hypodontia
- Johanson-Blizzard
- Kartagener
- Keipert
- Keutel
- KID
- Klippel-Feil
- Kniest
- LADD
- LEOPARD mandibulofacial dysotosis
- mannosidosis
- Marshall-Stickler syndrome
- MPS I, II, IV, VI
- mucosulfatidosis and multiple anterior dens invaginatus
- Nager
- oculo-auticulo-veterbral spectrum
- oral-facial-digital II
- osteogenesis imperfecta I–IV
- osteopathis striata
- osteopetrosis
- otodental
- otopalatodigital I and II
- Pallister-Killian
- postaxial acrofacial dysostosis
- premature aging and multiple nevi
- sclerosteosis
- Stickler
- symphalangism-brachydactyly syndrome
- Townes-Brock
- Van Buchem disease
- velocardiofacial
- Waardenburg
- Wildervanck

Source: Adapted from *Smith's Recognizable Patterns of Human Malformations* (6th ed.), by K. Jones, 2003. Philadelphia, PA: Saunders/Elsevier.

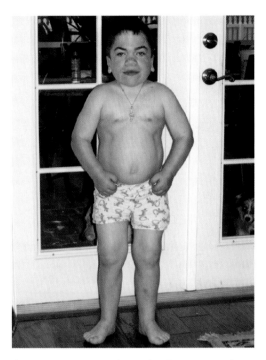

FIGURE 9–2. A child with Hunter syndrome. Note the coarsened facial features.

are easily recognized. Among the most striking are hypoplasia of the clavicles, which may allow an affected person to touch their shoulders in the midline, and supernumerary teeth, sometimes in excess of 50 secondary teeth.

■ Hearing impairment can also be a component of many different **inborn errors of metabolism**, such as biotinidase deficiency, Refsum disease, and 3-methylglutaconic aciduria. Most are associated with other findings, such as neurodevelopmental impairment, liver failure, and other organ dysfunction.

■ **Jervelle-Lange-Nielson syndrome** is an important deafness-related disorder because, although rare, it can be associated with sudden death. Affected persons have hearing impairment and long QT syndrome (LQTS), a disorder of cardiac conduction that predisposes to potentially fatal tachyarrhythmias. Jervelle-Lange-Nielson syndrome is autosomal recessive and is genetically heterogeneous, caused by mutations in either the gene *KCNQ1* (90%) or *KCNE1* (10%). It is important to remember that carriers of these mutations (e.g., parents of affected children) will have normal hearing, but may manifest LQTS, and therefore be at risk for fainting and sudden death. An evaluation by a cardiologist is therefore recommended.

■ Mutations in the **mitochondrial genome** typically cause a significant neurological neuromuscular disease. Examples include MELAS and MERRF syndromes (MELAS: mitochondrial myopathy, encephalopathy, lactic acidosis, and strokelike episodes; MERRF: myoclonus epilepsy associated with ragged-red fibers). However, other mutations in the mitochondrial genome may cause only hearing loss. One such example is the A1555G mutation that is associated with aminoglycoside toxicity (see section on nonsyndromic hearing impairment).

Other syndromic forms of hearing impairment have more clinical variability, so that detecting an affected individual may be very difficult. An affected individual may be so mildly affected that he or she may appear to have isolated hearing impairment. Examples include Waardenberg syndrome, Stickler syndrome, and branchio-oto-renal syndrome. To make the diagnosis, a detailed family history is essential, as other family members may manifest more classic symptoms.

■ **Waardenberg syndrome** is a group of disorders that share the common finding of sensorineural hearing impairment and segmental hypopigmentation that may involve the skin, hair, and/or eyes. There are several different subtypes that are distinguished by the presence of additional findings. Due to the clinical variability between and within subtypes, an affected individual may be very noticeable, manifesting a white forelock and distinct facial appearance (Figure 9–3); others will have no additional findings beyond hearing impairment, making it a very difficult diagnosis.

Individuals with Waardenberg syndrome type 1I manifest dystopia canthorum, a lateral displacement of the inner canthi, creating the appearance that the eyes are too far apart (Figure 9–4). About 60% of persons with Waardenberg syndrome type 1 have hearing impairment, which can be variable but is often bilateral and profound. Waardenberg syndrome type 1 is an autosomal dominant disorder caused by mutations in *PAX3*. Currently available genetic testing will detect over 90% of disease causing mutations in persons with Waardenberg syndrome type 1.

In Waardenberg syndrome type 2, dystopia canthorum is *not* present. The likelihood of severe hearing impairment is approximately 75%. Although Waardenberg syndrome type 2 is also autosomal dominant, it is caused by mutations in a different gene, *MITF*.

Waardenberg syndrome type 3 is very rare. Also called Klein-Waardenburg syndrome, it is a more severe variant of type 1. Affected individuals manifest facial findings of type 1, but also have limb anomalies and neural tube defects. Type 3 is autosomal recessive, caused by homozygosity for *PAX3* mutations. It typically is seen in areas of the world where there is a high rate of consanguinity.

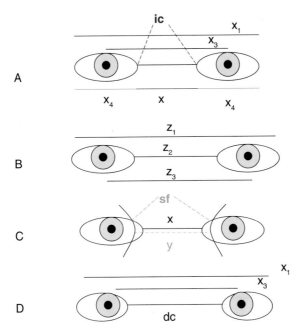

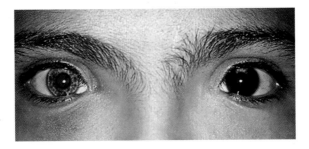

FIGURE 9–3. Eye spacing. **A.** Normal eye spacing, where the space between the inner canthi (IC), x, is the same as a palpebral fissure lengths (eye openings), x_2. **B.** Hypertelorism, with the inner canthal distance, z_2, outer canthal distance, z_1, and interpupillary distance, z_3, are all over the 95th centile. **C.** Telecanthus, with skin folds, *sf*, covering the inner canthi the eyes appear to widely, y, set but are actually normally spaced. This is often seen in Down syndrome, and other conditions with a flat nasal bridge, but can also be a normal variant in the general population. **D.** Dystopia canthorum, which is the eye finding in Waardenberg syndrome type 1. Here the interpupillary and outer canthal distances are approximately normal, but the inner canthi are laterally displaced, making that space (*dc*) too wide.

FIGURE 9–4. Dystopia canthorum and iris heterochromia. (Courtesy of Raoul C. M. Hennekam, ICH, London.)

Waardenberg syndrome type 4 also is very rare. It has the additional finding of Hirschsprung disease, a congenital deficiency of nerve cells in a segment of the colon that causes a blockage in the intestine, which is lethal if not corrected by surgery. Waardenberg syndrome type 4 is autosomal dominant, and is caused by mutations in the endothelin receptor B gene or the *SOX10* gene.

■ **Stickler syndrome**, also called hereditary arthro-ophthalmopathy, is a common autosomal dominant disorder that is characterized by significant vision problems and early onset arthritis. Affected individuals may have severe myopia and be at risk for retinal detachment, which can, if untreated, lead to blindness. Symptoms of arthritis may begin as early as the second decade of life, and can lead the requirement for joint replacement surgery in the third or fourth decade of life. There is radiographic evidence of a mild form of a skeletal disorder involving the joints and spine, called spondyloepiphyseal dysplasia. Other associated findings include midfacial underdevelopment, a small jaw, and cleft palate. It is the most common genetic syndrome that causes Pierre Robin sequence, a particular type of cleft palate caused by a small jaw (discussed in more detail in Chapter 10). More than 80% of affected individuals will manifest a mild hearing impairment, typically involving high-frequency sounds. Stickler syndrome may be caused by mutations in one of three different collagen genes: COL2A1, COL11A1, and COL11A2. Mutations in the COL11A2 gene are not associated with vision problems because COL11A2 is not expressed in the eye.

■ **Branchio-oto-renal (BOR) syndrome** is another autosomal dominant disorder that is very variable. The main clinical manifestations include branchial fistula or cysts (seen in about two-thirds of cases); hearing impairment, which can be mild to severe (89%); and renal anomalies (66%), which can range from clinically insignificant to lethal bilateral hypoplasia. BOR is caused by mutations in the genes *EYA1* and *SIY1*.

■ **Osteogenesis Imperfecta** is a group of disorders that are characterized by bones that fracture with minimal trauma (Table 9–3). Type II is lethal, as affected infants die in utero, or shortly after birth. Type III associated with fractures that heal with progressive deformation of the bones. Affected individuals fracture with even normal handling, and have significant long-term complications. Many die at an early age. Types I and IV are relatively milder. Affected individuals suffer fractures, but they heal normally, and long-term survival is typical. Complications include dentogenesis imperfecta (abnormally formed teeth), and hearing loss. This typically begins in the second decade of life as a conductive loss, although as it

TABLE 9–3. The Subtypes of Osteogenesis Imperfecta

Subtype	Features
Type 1	Normal stature, little or no skeletal deformity with healing fractures; all have blue sclerae; half will have hearing loss, few will have dentogenesis imperfecta
Type 2	Perinatal lethal; minimal skeletal ossification, beaded ribs, flat vertebrae.
Type 3	Progressive deforming. Many fractures that heal abnormally; short stature very common; sclerae are blue, but lighten with age; dentogenesis imperfecta and hearing loss are very common.
Type 4	Variable degree of fractures, with little or no deformity and short stature; normal sclerae, dentogenesis imperfecta very common, hearing loss not very common.

progresses there may be a sensorineural component as well. The hearing loss is primarily due to fixation of the ossicles, similar to what is seen in otosclerosis. The vast majority of osteogenesis imperfecta is autosomal dominant, caused by mutations in the genes for type I collagen, COL1A1 or COL1A2.

■ **Usher syndrome** is characterized by sensorineural hearing impairment and progressive vision loss due to retinitis pigmentosa. It is exceptionally heterogeneous, with three clinical subtypes. Usher syndrome type I is characterized by congenital and profound sensorineural hearing impairment accompanied by vestibular dysfunction. The latter is the defining characteristic of Usher type I, which causes affected children to be delayed in motor development skills like walking and sitting. Type II Usher syndrome does not manifest vestibular dysfunction, so the diagnosis may not be suspected until the onset of vision loss. Usher type III is characterized by postlingual progressive sensorineural hearing loss, later onset retinitis pigmentosa, and variable impairment of vestibular function.

Although all forms are inherited in an autosomal recessive manner, Usher syndrome demonstrates remarkable genetic heterogeneity. At least eight different genes can cause type I. Four can cause type II, but only one gene, *USH3,* has been found to cause type III.

■ **Pendred syndrome** is an autosomal recessive disorder often associated with congenital nonprogressive hearing impairment that is severe to profound. However the hearing loss can be postlingual and progressive. It is accompanied later in life by goiter (enlargement of the thyroid gland) that is usually not associated with thyroid dysfunction. A temporal bone CT scan will identify unilateral or bilateral dilated vestibular aqueducts or Mondini malformation (dilated vestibular aqueduct with cochlear hypoplasia). Pendred syndrome is caused by mutations in the gene *SLC26A4*. Mutation in *SCL26A4* also cause nonsyndromic hearing impairment as DFNB4, which is characterized by isolated uni- or bilateral Mondini malformation of dilated vestibular aqueduct

NONSYNDROMIC HEARING IMPAIRMENT

Nonsyndromic, or isolated, hearing impairment refers to hearing impairment that occurs without other medical problems. As discussed above, it is classified by age of onset, severity, and anatomic location. It is among the most genetically heterogeneous disorders. Current estimates are that over 120 different genes are involved in hearing. To date, more than 80 different genetic loci that contain hearing-related genes have been identified. For a more current figure, the reader is referred to the Hereditary Hearing Loss Home Page (http:///webhost.ua.ac.be/hhh/).

Understanding the nomenclature is necessary when considering the genetics of nonsyndromic hearing impairment (Table 9–4). DFNA refers to a genetic locus that causes autosomal dominant hearing impairment; DFNB refers to autosomal recessive; and DFN refers to an X-linked locus. There is no designation for mitochondrial inherited hearing impairment.

TABLE 9–4. Designation for Genetic Loci Associated with Nonsyndromic (Isolated) Hearing Impairment*

Autosomal dominant forms: **DFNA**
  ~22%, DFNA1-54

Autosomal recessive forms: **DFNB**
  ~77%, DFNB1-67

X-linked forms: **DFN**
  ~1%, DFN1-8

Y-linked forms: **DFNY**
  <1%, DFNY1

Maternal (mitochondrial) inheritance
  ~1%, 7 known mutations

---

*As of March 2006; see the Hereditary Hearing Loss homepage (http://webhost.ua.ac.be/hhh/) for more details.

With each hearing impairment-associated genetic locus, a number follows this designation. The loci are numbered in the order in which they were discovered by researchers. For example, "DFNB8" was the eighth autosomal recessive hearing impairment genetic locus identified. About 75 to 80% of genetically determined prelingual hearing impairment is inherited as an autosomal recessive trait. Autosomal dominant (20%), X-linked (2-5%), and mitochondrial (1%) forms make up the remainder. In contrast, the majority of later onset progressive hearing loss is autosomal dominant.

Furthermore, there is overlap with syndromic hearing impairment, as there are several genes that underlie both syndromic and nonsyndromic causes of hearing impairment. Examples include Myosin VIIA, which underlies Usher syndrome IB, DFNA11, and DFNB2; COL11A2 (Stickler syndrome and DFNA13), and FGFR3 (Muenke syndrome and DFNA6). There is also redundancy, instances in which two or more loci were assigned to the same gene. For example, WFS1 is DFNA6/14/38 (see below), an occurrence that arose because three research groups independently identified what appeared to be separate genetic loci that contained a hearing-impairment-related gene. These genetic loci were close, or even overlapping, but appeared to be distinct and were given separate designations. However, as the genetic map improved it was realized that these three apparently distinct loci contained the same hearing-related gene. Another example of this is *TECTA*, which was mapped as both DFNA8 and DFNA12.

Some genes also can cause both autosomal recessive and autosomal dominant hearing impairment. An example is Myosin VIIA, which can be mutated in DFNA11, DFNB2, and also cause one form of Usher syndrome, USH1B.

Gap Junction β 2 (the Connexin 26 gene)

Although there are over several dozen genes known to be involved in prelingual nonsyndromic hearing impairment, the most common by far is *GJβ2*, the gene that encodes Connexin 26 at the locus DFNB1. Connexins are proteins that make up connexons, gap junctions that facilitate the transport of small molecules and ions between cells. Connexin 26 is highly expressed in the cochlear duct, and may be involved in recycling potassium in the inner ear.

Mutations in *GJβ2* account for about 30% of severe-to-profound nonsyndromic prelingual hearing impairment in individuals of northern European descent, and more than 50% if the family history suggests autosomal recessive inheritance for the hearing impairment. It is also common in Israel and parts of Asia and Latin America as well. The carrier rate for a *GJβ2* mutation in Caucasians is about 3%, with one mutation, 35delG, accounting for almost two-thirds of cases. Different mutations are more common in other ethnic groups: 167delT is seen in about 4% of Ashkenazi Jews, while 235delC is seen in about 1% of Japanese. Interestingly, *GJβ2* mutations are not common in individuals of African descent.

There has been extensive research to correlate the exact genetic change in *GJβ2* with the level of hearing impairment. These studies are called genotype-phenotype correlations.

Some mutations, such as 35delG, cause no protein to be made, whereas others are associated with diminished protein function. Extensive and detailed studies have correlated the exact type of mutation with the degree of hearing impairment. For example, individuals with two (e.g., are homozygous) 35delG mutations typically have profound hearing impairment. The 35delG mutation has a severe effect on the gene, causing it to produce no Connexin 26 protein. Less severe mutations, such as M34T, are associated with the production of Connexin 26 that retains some function. Such mutations have been shown to cause less severe hearing impairment.

When widespread testing of *GJβ2* of hearing-impaired children began, it was noted that a larger than expected number were found to be carriers of a single mutation, 16% in some studies (compared to the expected rate of about 3% in the general population). Subsequently, many of these patients were found to have a deletion in a gene that is physically adjacent to *GJβ2* in the locus DFNB1, *GJβ6* (Connexin 30). Such individuals are termed "double heterozygotes," as they carry mutations involving two separate genes. Due to its high frequency, it is now common for labs to test for the *GJB6* deletion in a hearing-impaired subject if only one *GJβ2* mutations is found. Individuals with this complex genotype manifest the most severe level of hearing impairment seen with *GJβ2* mutations, even greater than that seen in individuals who are homozygous for the severe 35delG mutation. Although the reason for this is not yet known, it may be that the *GJβ6* deletion affects the expression of the "normal" *GJβ2*.

WFS1 AND AUTOSOMAL DOMINANT HEARING IMPAIRMENT

Mutations in the gene WFS1 (DFNA6/14/38) cause autosomal dominant sensorineural hearing impairment that is mild to moderate and bilaterally symmetrical. Initially, the hearing impairment is most evident at the low frequencies (primarily below 4000 Hz), giving WFS1-related hearing impairment an up-sloping pattern. However, the hearing impairment will progress, with largest progression being in the higher frequencies. This results in a flat audiogram by the fifth decade of life, with a leveling out at 50 to 70 dB.

Mutations in WFS1 also cause Wolfram syndrome, an autosomal recessive disease characterized by diabetes insipidus, diabetes mellitus, optic atrophy, and deafness giving rise to the acronym DIDMOAD for this disease. Remarkably, the hearing loss in DIDMOAD syndrome is in the high frequencies. The reason for the additional findings in DIDMOAD may be explained by the different types of mutations seen in each condition. For DIDMOAD, the WFS1 mutations tend to be severe, knocking out the gene's function, whereas those that cause nonsyndromic hearing impairment are less severe.

Audiogram patterns can provide an important clue to identifying the responsible gene or locus. Most hearing-impairment-related genes produce audiogram profiles that may not be unique, but can at least help narrow down the list of possible causative genes. WFS1 is one such example, as it is the most likely gene to test in a child with low-frequency hearing impairment. About 10% will have a WFS1 mutation, but the likelihood sharply rises to over 75% for those who have a family history of progressive hearing impairment. Looking at the audiologic profiles of affected individuals at different ages can also provide important information: they may have a similar up-sloping pattern early on, but the changes of the audiologic pattern may distinguish one genetic form from another.

OTHER HEARING-IMPAIRMENT-RELATED GENES

In addition to *GJβ2*, several dozen genes are known to be associated with hearing impairment. These include both autosomal recessive, autosomal dominant, X-linked, and even mitochondrial forms. However, none individually is as common as *GJβ2*, and therefore testing for the many of these genes is available only on a research basis. Table 9–5 provides a select list of the deafness-related genes that can be tested for commercially. For a more complete list, see http://www.genetests.org. This list is relatively small because establishing testing for an individual gene is an expensive proposition for a clinical lab, and therefore not viable if the volume of test requests is likely to be low. However, it is expected that advancing genetic testing technology will permit screening of multiple genes relatively easily.

TABLE 9–5. Deafness-Related Genes for Which Clinical Genetic Testing Is Available*

Autosomal Dominant

EYA1 encodes the protein Eyes Absent 1. Mutations or deletions in *EYA1* cause Branchio-oto-renal (BOR) syndrome. However, *EYA1* mutations are found in only 30% of BOR patients, so negative tests does not exclude BOR syndrome.

WFS1 (DFNA6/14) encodes the protein Wolframin. Mutations in *WFS1* cause a familial low-frequency hearing loss that can progress over time to involve all frequencies.

KCNQ4 **(DFNA2)** encodes a voltage-gated potassium channels that regulate electrical signaling and the ionic composition of biologic fluids in the inner ear.

continues

TABLE 9–5. *continued*

COCH (**DFNA9**) encodes an inner ear protein. Mutations in COCH cause an autosomal dominant hearing loss that can be associated with variable vestibular malfunction in some patients. Onset of hearing loss patients with DFNA9 occurred between 20 and 30 years of age, is initially more profound at high frequencies, and displayed variable progression to anacusis by 40 to 50 years of age.

Autosomal Recessive

GJβ2 (**DFNB1**) encodes the Connexin 26 protein. Mutations in *GJβ2* are the most common genetic cause of congenital hearing impairment. Testing should be done for any patient with congenital hearing impairment of any degree with a negative family history, or a history that suggests autosomal recessive inheritance. Testing for *GJβ2* typically includes screening for the associated deletion of the neighboring gene, *GJβ6*.

SLC26A4 (**DFNB4**) encodes the protein Pendrin. Mutations in *SLC26A4* cause Pendred syndrome, as well as a subset of hearing loss associated with either Mondini dysplasia or dilated vestibular aqueduct syndrome.

X-Linked

POU3F4 (**DFN3**) encodes a transcription factor, a gene whose product regulates the expression of other genes. Mutations in or near the POU3F4 gene cause deafness that can be conductive (due to impaired stapes mobility), and/or mixed with a superimposed sensorineural component that can be progressive.

Mitochiondrial

MTRNR1 encodes the mitochondrial 12S ribosomal RNA protein. Two different mutations in this gene, C1494T and A1555G, have been associated with hearing loss as a result of aminoglycoside exposure.

MTTS1 encodes the mitochondrial transfer RNA-serine protein. The A7445G mutation has been found in several families with maternally inherited, progressive, nonsyndromic sensorineural hearing loss.

MTTL1 encodes the mitochondrial transfer RNA-leucine protein. The A3243G mutation has been found in several families segregating maternally inherited diabetes mellitus and sensorineural hearing loss. The A3243G mutation also is found in MELAS (Myopathy, Encephalopathy, Lactic Acidosis, Strokelike Episodes), and in a small percentage of diabetics.

*More than 70 genes are known to be involved in hearing impairment. Clinical testing is available only for a small number. The list above was adopted from the Molecular Otolaryngology Laboratory at the Molecular Otolaryngology Research Laboratories at the University of Iowa (http://www.medicine.uiowa.edu/otolaryngology/MorlLab/). This list represents a very small percentage of known hearing-related genetic loci and genes. For a complete list please, and for more details, see the Hereditary Hearing Loss homepage (http://webhost.ua.ac.be/hhh/).

THE GENETICS OF AMINOGLYCOSIDE-RELATED HEARING LOSS

Aminoglycoside antibiotics are known to have an ototoxic effect. However, it is also known that not everyone exposed to even very high levels of these antibiotics loses their hearing. Recent research has revealed a genetic susceptibility that explains why some people lose their hearing after aminoglycoside exposure.

In studying a large family that segregated maternally inherited deafness (see Chapter 2), researchers identified a mutation in the mitochondrial 12sRNA gene, called A1555G. In further studies, it became clear that this mutation caused a very variable type of hearing loss—some carriers would lose their hearing slowly, beginning at any age, whereas other did not develop any hearing loss. Interestingly, further studies revealed that all mutation carriers who did develop hearing loss had been exposed to an aminoglycoside antibiotic. Although this mutation appears to be a common cause of aminoglycoside-induced hearing loss in some regions of the world, it is not common in the United States. However, it is very important to identify the presence of this mutation in any family that segregates maternally inherited hearing loss in order to prevent that child from receiving an aminoglycoside antibiotic, and therefore losing his or her hearing. Another mutation in the same gene, C1494T, has also been associated with aminoglycoside exposure.

OTOSCLEROSIS

Otosclerosis is the most common cause of hearing loss, being found in up to 1% of Caucasian adults. Hearing problems typically begin in the third to fourth decade and 90% of cases are diagnosed before age 50 years. It is caused by sclerosis of the ossicles in the inner ear, primarily at the stapedio-vestibular joint, resulting in a conductive hearing loss. This can be corrected by microsurgery, but there may also be a sensorineural loss as well. Microsurgery can correct the stapes fixation on the oval window and improve hearing. The etiology of otosclerosis is not known. It is clearly heterogeneous. A genetic basis seems evident for at least some cases, as autosomal dominant transmission has been reported, and several otosclerosis-related genetic loci have been mapped. One subset of otosclerosis is due to defects in type I collagen, the same gene involved in osteogenesis imperfecta. Sequelae to earlier measles infection has also been postulated as another possible cause.

GENETIC TESTING FOR HEARING IMPAIRMENT

The introduction of genetic testing for nonsyndromic hearing impairment has been rapid. As recently as the 1990s, genetics had little to offer. In an effort to determine causality for the hearing impairment, an evaluation would include a complete medical history to look for contributing causes (e.g., infection, prematurity); a family history to look for Mendelian segregation of hearing impairment; and a physical exam to look for subtle findings to suggest an underlying genetic syndrome. Often laboratory tests would be ordered as well, screening for possible causes such as hypothyroidism and congenital infection. If all was noncontributory, only inexact recurrence risk counseling could be offered. For example, hearing parents of a deaf child have a 1 in 6 chance of having another hearing-impaired child. This number is inexact for a given family, as it reflects the fact that different etiologic subtypes of isolated hearing impairment are indistinguishable. Today, genetic testing can offer more exact information, information that has implications beyond recurrence risk counseling. However, for patients and their families to gain the maximum benefit from the testing, it must be carried out in the proper manner, which includes pre- and post-test genetic counseling. Several groups have proposed algorithms for carrying out clinical genetic testing for hearing impairment.

The benefits of genetic testing include:

1. *Avoiding unnecessary and costly testing.* An infant or child with new diagnosis of hearing impairment often will have a battery of tests and evaluations ordered to establish the cause. The cost and inconvenience of these tests can be avoided in a substantial number of cases if mutation screening of *GJβ2* is ordered first.

2. *Defining recurrence risk.* Prior to genetic testing, recurrence risk counseling was based on pedigree structure. For example, normal-hearing parents of a deaf child have a 15 to 20% chance of having a second deaf child (Table 9–6). Because this information is derived from population studies, it cannot be applied to specific couples. In one family, for example, hearing impairment may be caused by a congenital infection; in another family it may be due to a recessively inherited genetic mutation. Each family has its own very different recurrence risks, and each is clearly different from the empiric population-based figures. However, unless these families can be distinguished, family-specific recurrence chance counseling is not possible. Today, genetic testing allows us, to a limited degree, to distinguish families, which will provide them with a very accurate recurrence figure. If a child tests positive for DFNB1-related deafness, for example, the parents' recurrence chance is 25% for each future pregnancy. Furthermore, prenatal testing also becomes an option when the specific genetic cause is identified.

TABLE 9–6. Empiric Recurrence Risk for Profound Childhood Sensorineural Hearing Impairment of Unknown Cause

Factor	Risk
Affected child	1/6
1 child, consanguinity	1/4
1 child, 2+ normal sibs	1/10
2 affected children	1/4
1 parent, 1 child	1/2
1 parent	1/20
Parent + parent's sibs	1/100
Sibs of parent, parent normal	<1/100

3. *Dispel incorrect notions of what caused the hearing impairment.* Parents often incorrectly assume that their child's hearing impairment was caused by a maternal exposure to a medication, or an environmental factor like loud noise. Others incorrectly believe that the hearing impairment is genetic because an older relative lost hearing later in life. These assumptions may lead to feelings of guilt as well as give parents an incorrect understanding of recurrence chances.

4. *Provide prognostic information.* Currently, genetic testing is used primarily to confirm a diagnosis or to assist in reproductive counseling. However, genetic testing also provides prognostic information in at least three areas. First, hearing impairment caused by *GJβ2* and/or *GJβ6* mutations is not associated with other medical problems and it is typically not progressive. Second, as stated above, it is possible to predict the severity of the hearing deficit based on the type of mutations present in *GJβ2*. A child with two mutations that completely knock-out the gene's function is typically associated with more severe hearing impairment than that seen in children with at least one more mild mutation. Third, the prognosis for children with *GJβ2*-related hearing impairment who undergo cochlear implantation is excellent with respect to language skills. It is hoped that, as we learn more about the clinical course of each genetic form of hearing impairment, habilitation plans may be tailored to the individual child based on specific genetic findings.

Even after a complete evaluation and genetic testing, an etiology will not be identified in many children. In this case, it important to have periodic re-evaluation, as new findings may develop that suggest a specific etiology. For example, the child's mother may learn that a male relative has nephritis, suggesting the need to consider testing for Alport syndrome, or the child may develop retinitis pigmentosa, a euthyroid goiter, or a prolonged QT interval, suggesting Usher, Pendred, or Jervell-Lange-Nielson syndromes, respectively. Even if no new findings emerge, repeating genetic testing in 2 to 5 years may be warranted, as genetic detection rates will increase with the use of new technologies like gene chips and microarray platforms that can test multiple genes at once. Such testing is expected in the not too distant future.

RECOMMENDED READING

Genetic Evaluation of Congenital Hearing Loss Expert Panel. American College of Medical Genetics. (2002). Genetics evaluation guidelines for the etiologic diagnosis of congenital hearing loss [Position statement]. *Genetic Medicine*, *4*(3), 162–171. This position statement was put forth by an expert panel convened by the American College of Medical Genetics, the largest society for clinical genetics. It reviews the role of genetics evaluation and genetic testing for the child with hearing impairment.

Hereditary Hearing Loss Home Page. (2007). Available at: http://webh01.ua.ac.be/hhh/ This Web site is intended for researchers and clinicians are involved in hearing impairment. It provides an up-to-date catalogue of genes and genetic loci involved in hearing impairment.

Robin, N. H., Prucka, S. K., Woolley, A., & Smith, R. H. J. (2005). Genetic testing as a component of the evaluation of the child with hearing impairment. *Current Opinion in Pediatrics*, *17*, 709–712. This paper proposes a cost-effective method for evaluating newborns with SNHI.

Smith, R. J., Bale, J. F., Jr., & White, K. R. (2005). Sensorineural hearing loss in children. *Lancet*, *365*(9462), 879–890. An excellent overview of SNHI.

Torello, H. V., Reardon, W., & Gorlin, J. (2004). *Hereditary hearing loss and its syndromes* (2nd ed.). Oxford: Oxford University Press.

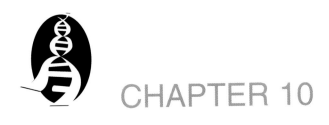

CHAPTER 10

Craniofacial Genetics I
Cleft Lip and Cleft Palate

*I*n this chapter, we review the genetic evaluation of orofacial clefting. As was the case in the previous chapter on hearing impairment, the first main point is to differentiate syndromic from nonsyndromic clefting. We then review several of the most common genetic syndromes that feature clefting as a common presenting manifestation, including velocardiofacial syndrome and Stickler syndrome. Finally, we review the genetic issues with nonsyndromic clefting, including genetic counseling and the present and future role for genetic testing.

OVERVIEW

Orofacial clefting—cleft lip with or without cleft palate or cleft palate alone—is a common and complex malformation. Affected children face a wide variety of medical issues and potential complications, extending beyond the surgical repair of the cleft. At every age, individuals with a cleft require evaluations and interventions by a wide variety of specialists. This care is best provided in the setting of a multidisciplinary cleft clinic. In this setting, many different health care providers can be seen in a single visit, including medical genetics. The overall composition and function of the multidisciplinary cleft team is discussed in more detail at the end of the chapter.

Genetics is an integral part of the multidisciplinary cleft clinic, as every affected child should be evaluated by a medical geneticist at some point. This evaluation has several goals. As was discussed for the child with hearing impairment, one major goal of the genetics evaluation for the child with a cleft is to determine if the cleft is an isolated anomaly or one finding in a child with a genetic syndrome. Some children, especially those with other major anomalies, such as a congenital heart defect, likely have already had a genetics evaluation and genetic testing. However, many patients, especially those with no other obvious abnormalities, may not have been seen by a geneticist. Furthermore, a re-evaluation is reasonable for older children who have seen a geneticist but no diagnosis was made but who now have additional findings, such as an unusual facial appearance or learning delays. Important findings may be absent or difficult to identify in an infant.

PREVALENCE

According to a recent Centers for Disease Control (CDC; 2006) report, orofacial clefting is now the most common birth defect in the United States, with about 6800 cleft babies born each year, a birth prevalence of about 1 in 600 overall. The frequency of orofacial clefting has risen in the past 10 years; however, there is no explanation for this rise.

Across the world, the prevalence of cleft lip with or without a cleft palate varies. It is most common among individuals of Asian descent and is least common among individuals of African ancestry, with the rate among Northern European Caucasians in between. Unlike cleft lip with or without a cleft palate, the prevalence of cleft palate alone is fairly constant in all ethnic groups, at about 1 per 1000. However, the frequency is greater if other forms of cleft palate are included beyond an overt gap in the soft palate, such as submucous cleft palate (where a mucosal lining covers the muscular gap in the soft palate), bifid uvula, or occult submucous cleft palate (Figure 10-1). Although less extensive than an overt cleft palate, these less obvious forms of cleft palate can still be associated with clinically significant palatal dysfunction, such as velopharyngeal insufficiency and speech problems that often require surgical correction.

Although they are often grouped together, cleft lip with or without a cleft palate is etiologically quite distinct from cleft palate alone (Table 10-1). Cleft lip with or without a cleft palate occurs twice as often in males, whereas cleft palate alone is twice as common in females. Conversely, cleft palate alone is twice as likely to be associated with other anomalies (20-60%) or be part of a genetic syndrome (25-40%) compared to cleft lip with or without a cleft palate (10-30% and 10-25%, respectively).

The fact they are different is also obvious when examining the embryology of these two defects (Figure 10-2A-E). Cleft lip occurs due to a failure of fusion of the median nasal prominence with the premaxillary process at about 42 days into gestation. Often the defect extends to the anterior hard palate, which is part of the same structure. This causes an intra-oral space that is too large to permit the lateral palatine processes to fuse and form the soft

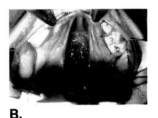

B.

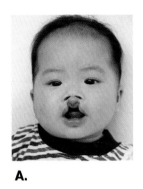

A.

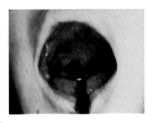

C.

FIGURE 10–1. **A.** Bilateral cleft lip and palate. **B.** Cleft palate **C.** Bifed uvula. (10–1B and 10–1C, Courtesy of Dr. Robert J. Shprintzen.).

TABLE 10–1. Differences Between Cleft Lip With or Without a Cleft Palate (CLP) and Cleft Palate Alone (CPA)

Feature	CLP	CPA
Incidence and prevalence varies by race	Yes	No
Male to female ratio	2/1	1/2
Rate of associated malformations	8–28%	22–61%
Likelihood of an underlying syndrome	10–25%	25–40%

palate starting at about 63 days gestation, resulting in a cleft palate as well. It is easy to understand then, how an insult that causes a cleft lip may also result in a cleft palate. However, it should also be apparent that an insult that causes a cleft palate could not be associated with a cleft lip, as the lip has already formed by the point at which the cleft palate occurs.

One important implication of this is that couples who have a child with a cleft palate are at increased risk for having another child with a cleft palate, but *not* a cleft lip or cleft lip and palate. Similarly, for parents of a baby with a cleft lip and palate, their risk for future offspring is for cleft lip, cleft lip and palate, but *not* cleft palate alone. This is true not only for isolated clefts, but for those seen as part of a genetic syndrome as well.

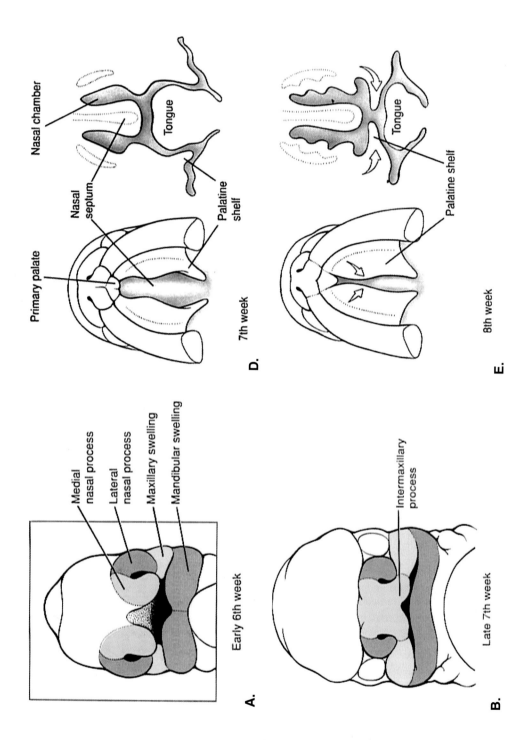

Medial nasal process
Lateral nasal process
Maxillary swelling
Mandibular swelling

A.

Early 6th week

Intermaxillary process

B.

Late 7th week

Nasal chamber

Nasal septum

Primary palate

Tongue

Palatine shelf

D.

7th week

Tongue

Palatine shelf

E.

8th week

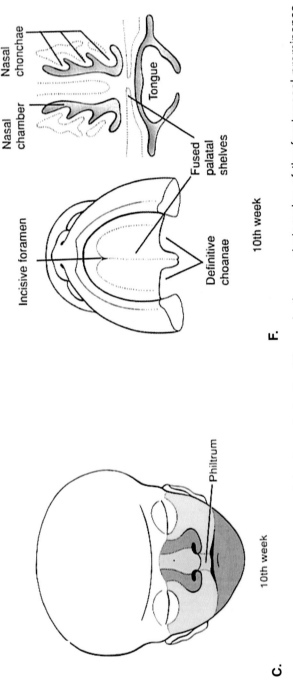

C.

Philtrum

10th week

F.

Incisive foramen

Definitive choanae

Fused palatal shelves

Nasal chamber

Nasal chonchae

Tongue

10th week

FIGURE 10–2. Development of the face. **A.** In the 6th week, the nasal placodes of the frontonasal prominence invaginate to form the nasal pits and the lateral and medial nasal processes. **B.** In the 7th week, the medial nasal processes fuse at the midline to form the intermaxillary process. **C.** By the 10th week, the intermaxillary process forms the philtrum of the upper lip. The dotted lines in D, E, and F represent regions of fusion of facial primordial. Formation of the secondary palate and nasal septum. The secondary palate forms from palantine shelves that grow medially from the maxillary swellings. During the same period, growth of the nasal septum separates the left and right nasal passages. The palatine shelves at first grow inferiorly on either side of the tongue (**D**) but then rapidly rotate upward to meet in the midline (**E**) where they fuse with each other and with the inferior edge of the nasal septum (**F**). (A–F reprinted with permission from *Human Embryology,* by W. J. Larsen, pp. 329, 331. Copyright 1993 Churchill-Livingstone).

However, certain syndromes do have both cleft lip with or without cleft palate and cleft palate alone as clinical features. Therefore, if you encounter a family in which some members have cleft palate alone (including submucous clefts) and other first-degree relatives (children, parents, or siblings) have cleft lip with or without cleft palate, it is possible that the family shares the same syndrome. The most common example of this is Van der Woude syndrome. This autosomal dominant disorder is characterized by the occurrence of cleft lip, cleft palate, and lip pits. Lip pits are accessory openings of the salivary glands, and therefore may secrete mucus (Figure 10–3). They are typically bilateral, and may be located anywhere on the buccal mucosa. For that reason, it is important to carefully inspect this region in every patient with an apparently isolated cleft because the recurrence risk counseling is significantly different. An individual with van der Woude syndrome has a 50% risk of passing on the mutant gene to an offspring, who may manifest clefting, which is far higher than the approximately 1 to 5% risk with nonsyndromic clefting.

Van der Woude syndrome is caused by mutations in the gene *interferon regulatory factor 6* (*IRF6*), located on chromosome 1q32. In some instances, Van der Woude syndrome is caused by a microdeletion of this chromosomal region. These patients also manifest mental retardation, presumably due to the fact that the deleted segment includes other genes in addition to IRF6, genes that are important in cognition.

Aside from the lip pits, a cleft caused by an IRF6 mutation is indistinguishable from a cleft caused by any other reason. It is not surprising then that *IRF6* mutations have been described as a common genetic cause of nonsyndromic clefting. Interestingly, different mutations in IRF6 cause a very different disorder, popliteal pterygium syndrome. This autosomal dominant disorder is also characterized by mixed types of clefting and lip pits, but affected individuals also have intra-oral fibrous bands, genital anomalies, and limb defects.

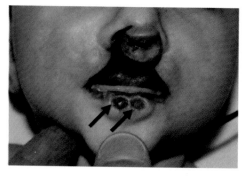

FIGURE 10–3. Lip pits, suggestive of Van der Woude syndrome. (Courtesy of John H. Grant, M.D.)

THE MANY CAUSES OF CLEFTING

Clefting is etiologically heterogeneous. IRF6 is only one of many genes that are associated with clefting, and there are many nongenetic causes as well. Although most clefting occurs as an isolated birth defect, in a significant percentage of cases, clefting is but one finding in a child with a genetic syndrome. There are several hundred multiple congenital anomaly syndromes that include clefting as one component of manifestation. Some clefting syndromes are caused by chromosomal imbalance—a duplication or deletion, but most are single genes disorders, inherited as autosomal dominant, autosomal recessive, or X-linked traits. For most, no genetic test is available, so they must be diagnosed by clinical evaluation. A detailed discussion of even a small number of these syndromes is beyond the scope of this chapter. Interested readers are referred to the reference texts listed at the end of the chapter, especially *Syndromes of the Head and Neck* (Gorlin, Cohen, & Hennekam, 2001).

Although many syndromes are readily identified due to their obvious anomalies, two of the most common syndromic forms of clefting have a much more subtle appearance and are, therefore, often missed.

Deletion 22q11 Syndrome
(Velocardiofacial Syndrome, Di George Syndrome)

Deletion 22q11 syndrome (del22q11) is among the most common genetic syndromes, with a birth prevalence estimated at between 1 in 2000 to 4000. It is the most common syndromic form of clefting. Although about 30% of affected children manifest an overt cleft palate, and nearly all of the remainder have palatal dysfunction due to a submucous cleft palate, occult submucous cleft palate, or a palate and pharynx that are anatomically intact but function poorly due to neuromuscular weakness. Furthermore, many patients have cognitive limitations that manifest as expressive language deficits. Therefore, nearly all affected individuals have speech and language problems.

Del22q11 is among the most clinically variable syndromes known. Owing to its wide variability, several conditions have been described as distinct entities that have subsequently been found to be due to the chromosome 22q11 deletion. Although they are often still referred to by their original names, we now know that they represent variable manifestations of del22q11, different points in the continuum of this disorder. Examples include DiGeorge syndrome, velocardiofacial (Shprintzen) syndrome, and conotruncal anomaly-face syndrome.

Over 180 different anomalies have been seen with del22q11, involving every organ system (Table 10–2). Despite this incredible clinical variation, the syndrome does have certain characteristic findings, including the palatal anomalies; conotruncal congenital heart defects (e.g., tetralogy of Fallot);

TABLE 10–2. A List of Select Findings from the Over 180 That Have Been Associated with Deletions of Chromosome 22q11.2

Craniofacial/Oral Findings

1. Overt, submucous or occult submucous cleft palate
2. Retrognathia (retruded lower jaw)
3. Platybasia (flat skull base)
4. Asymmetric crying facies in infancy
5. Structurally asymmetric face
6. Functionally asymmetric face
7. Vertical maxillary excess (long face)
8. Congenitally missing teeth
9. Small teeth
10. Enamel hypoplasia (primary dentition)
11. Hypotonic, flaccid facies
12. Downturned oral commissures
13. Cleft lip (uncommon)
14. Microcephaly

Eye Findings

15. Tortuous retinal vessels
16. Suborbital congestion ("allergic shiners")
17. Narrow palpebral fissures
18. Iris coloboma (uncommon)
19. Retinal coloboma (uncommon)
20. Small eyes
21. Mild orbital hypertelorism
22. Puffy upper eyelids

Ear/Hearing Findings

23. Overfolded helix
24. Attached lobules
25. Protuberant, cup-shaped ears
26. Small ears
27. Mild conductive hearing loss
28. Sensorineural hearing loss

Nasal Findings

29. Prominent nasal bridge
30. Bulbous nasal tip
31. Narrow nasal passages

Cardiac Findings

32. VSD (ventricular septal defect)
33. ASD (atrial septal defect)
34. Tetralogy of Fallot
35. Right-sided aorta
36. Truncus arteriosus
37. Interrupted aorta, type B
38. Coarctation of the aorta
39. Aortic valve anomalies
40. Aberrant subclavian arteries
41. Vascular ring
42. Anomalous origin of carotid artery

Vascular Anomalies

43. Medially displaced internal carotid arteries
44. Tortuous, kinked, absent, or accessory internal carotids
45. Jugular vein anomalies
46. Absence of vertebral artery (unilateral)
47. Low bifurcation of common carotid
48. Tortuous or kinked vertebral arteries
49. Circle of Willis anomalies

Neurologic and Brain Findings

50. Small cerebellar vermis
51. Cerebellar hypoplasia/dysgenesis
52. White matter hyperintensities
53. Generalized hypotonia
54. Cerebellar ataxia

TABLE 10–2. *continued*

55. Polymicrogyria
56. Spina bifida/meningomyelocele
57. Mild development delay
58. Enlarged Sylvian fissure

Problems in Infancy

59. Feeding difficulty, failure-to-thrive
60. Gastroesophageal reflux
61. Nasal regurgitation
62. Chronic constipation (usually not Hirschsprung megacolon)

Speech/Language

63. Severe hypernasality
64. Severe articulation impairment
65. Language impairment (usually mild delay)
66. Velopharyngeal insufficiency (usually severe)
67. Dyspraxia
68. High-pitched voice
69. Hoarseness

Cognitive/Learning

70. Learning disabilities (math concept, reading comprehension)
71. Concrete thinking, difficulty with abstraction
72. Drop in I.Q. scores in school years (test artifact)
73. Borderline normal intellect
74. Occasional mild mental retardation
75. Attention deficit hyperactivity disorder

Miscellaneous Anomalies

76. Bernard-Soulier disease
77. Juvenile rheumatoid arthritis

Psychiatric/Psychological

78. Bipolar affective disorder
79. Manic depressive illness and psychosis
80. Rapid or ultrarapid cycling of mood disorder
81. Mood disorder
82. Depression
83. Hypomania
84. Schizoaffective disorder
85. Impulsiveness
86. Flat affect
87. Dysthymia, cyclothymia
88. Schizophrenia
89. Social immaturity
90. Obsessive compulsive disorder
91. Generalized anxiety disorder
92. Phobias

Immunologic

93. Frequent upper and lower respiratory infections
94. Reduced T-cell populations

Genitourinary

95. Hypospadias
96. Cryptorchidism
97. G-U reflux

Endocrine

98. Hypocalcemia
99. Hypoparathyroidism
100. Hypothyroidism
101. Mild growth deficiency, relative small stature
102. Absent, hypoplastic thymus

Source: Modified from Robin and Shprintzen (2006).

a typical facial appearance; and a wide spectrum of learning disabilities; and psychiatric problems. As is the case with many genetic syndromes, the facial appearance in del22q11 is distinctive (Figure 10-4). However, the distinctive features are very subtle, and are often not appreciated by an untrained eye (e.g., anyone other than an experienced medical geneticist). The facial characteristics include narrow palpebral fissures, flat cheeks, a small mouth with sharp down-turned corners, small ears, and small teeth with dysplastic enamel.

Learning disabilities are nearly ubiquitous in del22q11. Although the IQ is often in the low normal range, the majority of cases have borderline or mildly retarded IQ scores. Behavioral problems include social immaturity, concrete thinking, obsessive compulsive traits, and attention deficit hyperactivity disorder. Finally, about one third of individuals with del22q11 will manifest a psychiatric disorder. Although many psychiatric disorders can be seen, the most common are affective disorders and schizophrenia. Del22q11 is the most common known genetic cause of psychiatric disease.

As seen in Table 10-2, the list of the potential anomalies seen with this disorder is extensive. The type of problem and age of diagnosis largely determines what syndrome name the patient receives. For example, a newborn with a conotruncal congenital heart defect, hypocalcemia, and immune dysfunction would be labeled "DiGeorge syndrome," whereas a child who presents later in life with hypernasal speech and learning problems would be labeled "velocardiofacial syndrome" or "Shprintzen syndrome." Finally, many deletion carriers are diagnosed only after the birth of a more classically affected child. About 10 to 15% of cases demonstrate such autosomal dominant transmission, and because of the wide clinical variability, it is prudent to test both

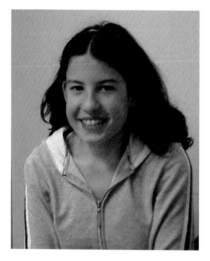

FIGURE 10-4. A 15-year-old girl with the classic facial characteristics of del22q11 syndrome.

parents of a newly diagnosed child. The reason for this clinical variability is not known. Remarkably, extensive variability can occur even among members of the same family.

The chromosomal deletion is most often not detectable on routine chromosome analysis. For that reason, specific FISH testing is often required (see Figure 6-4 in Chapter 6). This testing is often ordered liberally, which can at times be a danger, as a negative test can often incorrectly be assumed to rule out all genetic causes of cleft palate. Several other genetic syndromes, such as Kabuki syndrome (Figure 10-5) can be mistaken for del22q11. Therefore, repeat evaluation is recommended for patients who are suspected to have del22q11, but testing does not detect a deletion.

Stickler Syndrome and Pierre Robin Sequence

Stickler syndrome is another common syndromic cause of clefting that is often missed due to its relatively mild facial appearance (Figure 10-6). Most affected children have a relatively normal appearance, with only mild underdevelopment of the "midface" (cheeks, upper jaw). As discussed in more detail in Chapter 11, the main clinical manifestations of this autosomal dominant disorder include eye and vision problems (high myopia, risk for retinal detachment), early onset arthritis, and high-frequency sensorineural hearing impairment. Cleft palate is common as well, but although "typical" (e.g., "V-shaped") cleft palate can be seen), many cases of cleft palate in Stickler syndrome are associated with micrognathia as part of the Pierre Robin sequence. With Pierre Robin sequence, the gap in the palate is rounder, often referred to as "U-shaped."

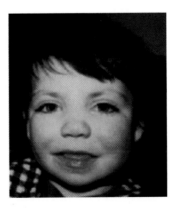

FIGURE 10–5. A child with Kabuki syndrome. (Reprinted with permission from "Array Based CGH and FISH Fail to Confirm Duplication of 8p22-23.1 in Association with Kabuki Syndrome," by Ming et al., 2005. *Journal of Medical Genetics, 42,* 49–53.)

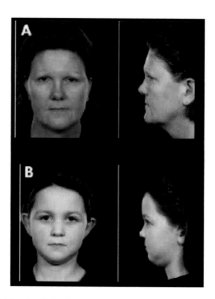

FIGURE 10–6. Stickler syndrome. Note the flat midface and nasal bridge and small mandible (Reprinted with permission from "Clinical Features of Type 2 Stickler Syndrome," by Paulson et al., 2004. *Journal of Medical Genetics*, 41, 107.)

In fact, Stickler syndrome is the most common genetic cause of Pierre Robin sequence, accounting for about 25% of all cases.

Pierre Robin sequence deserves special mention, as it is a genetically distinct form of clefting. It is often mistakenly referred to as "Pierre Robin syndrome," but it is not, in fact, a syndrome. Rather, it is a sequence—a series of anomalies derived from a single anomaly. During development, the mandible is too small, displacing the tongue superiorly, interfering with palatal closure at approximately 9 weeks gestation. Therefore, the cleft palate is not caused by an intrinsic problem with palatal closure, but is due to the small mandible.

As with any other sequence, a portion of Pierre Robin sequence occurs as part of a genetic syndrome. For Pierre Robin sequence, about half occurs as part of a syndrome, with Stickler syndrome being the most common, followed by del22q11. For that reason, it is recommended that every newborn with Pierre Robin sequence have a chromosome analysis and FISH testing for the chromosome 22q11 deletion, and an eye exam looking for the typical findings of Stickler syndrome. However, as one form of Stickler syndrome does not have eye involvement, patients with a normal eye exam should still be followed for other later manifestations of Stickler syndrome, such as mild spondyloepiphyseal dysplasia, hearing impairment, and early onset arthritis.

THE IMPORTANCE OF THE PREMAXILLA

The premaxillary segment is the space between the philtral columns, above the upper lip (Figure 10-7). Identifying this landmark is among the most important first steps when examining a child with a cleft lip. Normally, the premaxilla appears to "hang" free in children with a bilateral cleft lip. Hypoplasia, or absence of this segment, is suggestive of holoprosencephaly, a disorder of brain development characterized by a failure of the two cerebral hemispheres to normally separate (Figures 10-8A, 10-8B, and 10-8C). Other associated findings include eyes that are too close together ("hypotelorism") and a flat nose that may have only a single nostril. Some cases are caused by chromosomal abnormalities, such as trisomy 13, and these have other associated extracranial anomalies, such as congenital heart defects and renal dysplasia. However, about half of holoprosencephaly cases are caused by mutations in a single gene, such as *sonic hedgehog*. These cases typically manifest only brain and craniofacial abnormalities. Occasionally, these cases come to a cleft clinic for treatment, as the referring physician has not appreciated the abnormal facial findings and believes the child has an isolated cleft. As the prognosis for holoprosencephaly is exceptionally poor, many people will only do a cosmetic repair, if they operate at all. The genetic issues are, however, far more complex, and beyond the scope of this book. The key issue is to identify this type of cleft by the absence of the premaxillary segment, and to make the appropriate referral to a geneticist for evaluation and counseling for this severe birth defect.

The Genetics of Nonsyndromic Clefting

That genetic factors play a role in nonsyndromic clefting has been recognized for centuries. However, unlike what is seen with genetic syndromes, nonsyndromic clefting does not follow a simple Mendelian inheritance pattern. It is

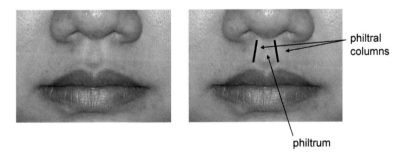

FIGURE 10–7. A normal philtrum, which is derived from the premaxillary segment. Shallow and/or abnormal philtrum is seen in many genetic syndromes.

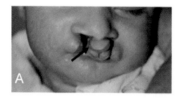
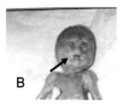
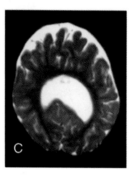

FIGURE 10–8. Two children with bilateral cleft lip and palate. Note the intact premaxillary segment (*arrow*) in **A**, whereas that structure is absent in **B**, suggesting the presence of an underlying brain malformation, holoprosencephaly. Note the single cerebral ventricle in **C**.

clear that genetic factors do not by themselves alone cause a cleft to occur. Nonsyndromic clefting is viewed as a multifactorial trait, one in which environmental and genetic factors interact to produce the phenotype. Clefting follows a threshold model, in which the liability (the combined effect of genetic and environmental factors) exceeds a given threshold, and the abnormal phenotype occurs (Figure 10-9). The magnitude of the genetic contribution to clefting has been debated. Early estimates placed it at 10 to 20%, but more recent data suggest that the genetic contribution is as high as 50%.

In the past few years, we have seen an explosion in our understanding of the genetic basis of nonsyndromic clefting. Mutations in several genes, including *MSX1*, *TBX22*, and *IRF6* have been identified in nonsyndromic cleft lip and cleft palate alone patients (Table 10-3). These discoveries have not, however, reached the point where they are clinically useful for all patients with nonsyndromic clefts. For that reason, the current genetic assessment of clefting remains limited to distinguishing syndromic from nonsyndromic cases, and, for nonsyndromic cases, quoting empirically deduced recurrence risks for parents of the affected child. For example, a clinical geneticist would counsel the unaffected parents of a child with a nonsyndromic cleft palate that they have approximately a 1% risk for having a child with a cleft palate with each future pregnancy. However, this recurrence risk figure is empiric, derived from large population studies that include cleft palate patients of many etiologic subtypes. It is the hope and expectation that genetic advances will lead

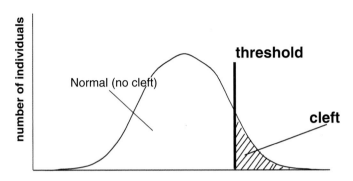

FIGURE 10–9. The "liability" is comprised of both genetic and nongenetic factors when their sum exceeds the threshold, the disease (e.g., cleft) occurs.

TABLE 10–3. Health Care Personnel in a Typical Cleft Clinic

Clinic Director*	Orthodontists
Clinic Coordinator (assistant to the clinic director)	Otorhinolaryngologists (ENT)
	Pediatrician
Audiologists	Pediatric Anesthesiologists
Craniofacial Surgeon	Pediatric Dentists and Prosthodontists
Geneticist	Pediatric Radiologists
Neurosurgeons	Physical Therapists
Nurses	Plastic Surgeons
Occupational Therapists	Speech-Language Pathologists
Oral and Maxillofacial Surgeons	Surgeon's Assistant

*The clinic director can be any member of the team. There is no single model, but the most common is for the director to be the clinic's pediatrician or one of the craniofacial surgeons.

to clinically useful genetic testing, and that this will provide an additional level of differentiation beyond what is possible by clinical evaluation only.

Currently, we are very limited in our assessment of the patient with a nonsyndromic cleft. A cleft that occurred due to a *TBX22* mutation may look no different than that associated with an *MSX1* or *IRF6* mutation, or one that is caused principally by environmental factors, such as maternal smoking. However, each type carries a different recurrence risk for the family: a cleft due to a mutation in *IRF6*, *TBX22* or *MSX1* will carry a higher recurrence risk than a cleft that was caused principally by an environmental factor, or by chance. Once we are able to differentiate these subtypes by genetic testing, we will be able to provide more accurate recurrence risk counseling than we can today. Furthermore, it is hoped that the ability to genetically subtype clefts will also provide prognostic information that can be used to guide medical management. It may be that the different genetic forms of clefting respond to surgery and therapies differently, with higher or lower complication rates.* For example, it may be that clefts caused by *MSX1* have a higher rate of maxillary underdevelopment, or that those due to *IRF6* generally require only minimal rate of residual velopharyngeal insufficiency. If this proves true, knowing the genetic subtype of a cleft patient will allow for more individualized surgical planning and therapies to better address the patient's specific risks.

THE MULTIDISCIPLINARY CLEFT TEAM

Children with cleft lip and/or cleft palate face a wide variety of medical issues and medical complications during their lives, requiring evaluations and interventions by a wide variety of specialists. As discussed above, to receive the best care possible, individuals with CLP should be seen in the setting of a multidisciplinary cleft clinic, where as many as a dozen different specialists can be seen in a single visit. This is both convenient for parents as well as the primary care providers, who can receive one concise letter that summarizes the team evaluation.

With the vast array of health care specialists, the multidisciplinary cleft clinic may seem mystifying and intimidating not only to parents but to the specialists in the clinic. Many are in unfamiliar fields, each evaluating and prescribing focused therapies.

The most critical aspect for the early management of a newborn with a cleft lip and/or palate is to ensure adequate feeding and nutrition (see Clefts and Breast Feeding). Therefore, the first cleft team member to evaluate the child is often a feeding specialist, most commonly a speech pathologist. This may be done at the first visit to the cleft clinic, or in the immediate newborn period while the baby is still in the hospital. Cleft infants are at risk for feeding difficulties due to the interruption of the baby's seal on the nipple (with a cleft lip), and the loss in the strength of the suck (with a cleft palate). As a consequence, babies with clefts often fatigue before they get the needed volume. The speech pathologist will recommend a special bottle and nipple, and educate the family in feeding techniques, as well as the warning signs for potential problems. The speech pathologist will work with the child and family on an ongoing basis. Problems may arise at any time, but especially after surgical repairs, and at the times when foods are advanced. Although most

---

*This has already been found to be the case with some forms of craniosynostosis (see Chapter 11).

Clefts and Breast Feeding

The notion that breast feeding is considered optimal for infants is widely accepted. Not only is breast milk the optimal source of nutrition for infants, breast-feeding also promotes mother-child bonding. Parents often ask about breast-feeding when they learn that their newborn has a cleft. For babies with a cleft lip and intact palate, breast feeding is not only possible, but may even be advantageous, as the soft breast tissue works as a mold to seal the cleft lip and promote suction. However, breast-feeding is more difficult in infants with a cleft of the palate, whether isolated or accompanying a cleft lip. With cleft palate, it is not likely adequate suction can be achieved. Breast feeding may be attempted, but it is likely that the baby will not be able to get an adequate volume of breast milk, and he or she may choke as the milk escapes from the mouth into the nasal passages. This is not dangerous to the nasal mucosa, as breast milk is not an irritant. However, there is the small risk of aspiration, which is obviously a more concerning potential complication. In such cases, infants with a cleft palate can still enjoy the benefits of breast milk given via bottle feeds that use specialized nipples.

children will adapt to spoon feeding and solid foods without difficulty, some require additional help in making this transition.

Other professionals who typically see an infant with a cleft include an audiologist, geneticist, and plastic surgeon. As discussed above, the geneticist's role is to determine the cause of the cleft (syndromic or nonsyndromic) and to counsel the family. Hearing loss is common for children with a cleft due to middle ear disease, so their hearing usually is tested by an audiologist at each visit.

The team's reconstructive surgeon often is team leader. Depending on the institution, this may be a plastic surgeon, an oral surgeon, or otolaryngologist. The surgeon will not only discuss his or her role, but also provide an overview of the clinic for the parents. At this initial visit, they will also take this time to discuss the surgical procedures that the child is facing. Primary procedures are those that address the anatomic defect, such as closure of the cleft lip or cleft palate; secondary procedures are those directed at correcting residual problems, or complications from the primary operations, such as a palatal fistula. Although most children with clefts will need several operations, the exact number depends on several variables. Some can be predicted by the extent of the defect (e.g., a bilateral cleft lip and palate will require more procedures compared to a unilateral cleft lip); others are more difficult to predict, such as the likelihood of residual speech problems or orthodontic complications.

For children with a cleft lip, the initial repair ("cheiloplasy") typically occurs at 10 to 12 weeks. However, timing may be altered if there are associated medical conditions, such as a cardiac malformation or poor nutrition. A cleft palate is typically repaired at 6 to 12 months. Earlier repair may result in better speech outcomes but more severe dental problems, whereas later repairs may be associated with improved maxillary growth and better dental occlusion, but less favorable speech outcomes. The choice of 6 to 12 months represents a balance between these two interests.

However, regardless of the surgeon's technique, experience, or any other variable, about 10% of cases will manifest postsurgical velopharyngeal insufficiency. That number is greater if there is an underlying genetic syndrome, such as del22qll. The speech-language pathologist's role is to monitor for speech problems, such as disorders of articulation and resonance. This can be done through simple screening tests, but more detailed diagnostic tools may be required.

The second major goal of surgery is to facilitate normal facial growth. This requires proper reconstruction of the facial muscles, as their normal activity stimulates primary and secondary growth centers of the facial skeleton. Abnormally oriented facial musculature, such as that seen in patients with clefts, will produce abnormal stimulation resulting in dental malocclusion, cross bites, impacted teeth, midface deficiency, nasal obstruction, and even apnea. However, even with the best repair, about 25% of cleft patients will have some residual deformities. These can be addressed with orthodontic measures, such as bracing, or may be more involved. Extensive surgery, such as a maxillary osteotomy, typically is not done until the facial skeletal growth is complete, usually the age of menarche for girls and about age 18 years for boys. Such orthodontic concerns are a dominant issue as patients with clefts age.

Hearing loss due to otitis media with middle ear effusion is present in virtually all infants under 2 years of age with unrepaired cleft palate. Repair of the cleft palate reduces the rate of otitis media, but myringotomy tubes are often placed to clear any effusions and, therefore, avoid hearing loss. Because even intermittent hearing loss can have a deleterious effect on speech and language development, and therefore academic achievement, it is crucial for all children with cleft palate to have frequent hearing evaluations by an audiologist. Although this problem decreases with age, for most patients, middle ear disease remains an important problem into adult life.

The long-term health of patients with clefts has been poorly studied. Most assume that, because clefts are a repairable birth defect, and the associated medical issues are for the most part readily treatable, these individuals should have normal long-term health. However, individuals with clefting have been shown to have a higher than expected incidence of psychiatric and behavioral diseases, an increased risk for cancer, and an increased mortality in general from all major causes of death. There is no explanation for these findings, as they are not related to coexisting birth defects or genetic syndromes. Although these findings must be confirmed by additional studies, they emphasize that clefting is a condition with long-term health concerns.

REFERENCES

Gorlin, R. J., Cohen, M. M., & Hennekam, R. C. (2001). *Syndromes of the head and neck* (4th ed., chaps. 20, 21, 22). Oxford, UK: Oxford University Press.

Centers for Disease Control and Prevention. (2006, January 6). *Morbidity and Mortality Weekly*, *54*(51–52), 1302–1305.

RECOMMENDED READINGS

Larson, W. J. (1993). *Human embryology* (chap. 12). London, UK: Churchill Livingstone.

Murphy, K. C., & Scambler, P. J. (2005). *Velo-cardio-facial syndrome.* Cambridge, UK: Cambridge University Press

Robin, N. H., Baty, H., Franklin, J., Guyton, F.C., Mann, J., et al. (2006). The multidisciplinary evaluation and management of cleft lip and palate [Review]. *Southern Medical Journal*, *99*(10), 1111–1120.

Stevenson, R. E., & Hall, J. G. (2006). *Human malformations and related anomalies* (2nd ed., Pt. 4, chap. 12). Oxford, UK: Oxford University Press.

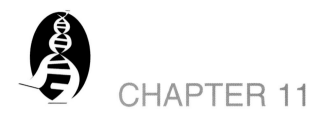

CHAPTER 11

Craniofacial Genetics II

Craniosynostosis and Related Syndromes

*I*n this final chapter we review the genetics of syndromes with prominent craniofacial findings. The first section focuses on craniosynostosis and its related syndromes; the second section is comprised of a number of brief reviews on a select group of genetic syndromes that have craniofacial findings. Most major pediatric medical centers have multidisciplinary clinics that are dedicated to the care of children with congenital craniofacial anomalies. Often these are combined with cleft clinics (see Chapter 10), as these patients need the same medical specialists. Although the types of anomalies seen in craniofacial clinics are limited to the craniofacial region, the variety is extensive, posing many complex medical and surgical challenges. Many children have additional anomalies beyond the craniofacial region, and many if not most have a genetic basis. This includes children with a single isolated anomaly as well. The role of the geneticist in these clinics is vital, as several hundred genetic syndromes have craniofacial findings as one manifestation. For many of these syndromes, the genetic basis is known, and testing is available. Some are relatively common; others are very rare. However, as discussed in Chapter 4, making a correct genetic diagnosis is crucial to providing the best medical care to the child and the most accurate information to the child's family. In this chapter, we review the genetic evaluation of the child with an abnormal head shape, including syndromic and nonsyndromic craniosynostosis, as well as a select number of common genetic syndromes with prominent craniofacial findings.

CRANIOSYNOSTOSIS AND ABNORMAL SKULL SHAPE

Craniosynostosis refers to the premature closure of one or more of the cranial sutures, the unossified membranes that bridge the bony plates of the developing fetal and infant skull (Figure 11–1). These sutures are the sites of skull growth, which occurs in response to the growth of the underlying brain and is quite rapid in the first few years of life. Skull growth is normally perpendicular to the plane of a cranial suture, but this is not possible if a cranial suture closes prematurely. This results in an abnormal skull shape, the exact nature of the shape determined by the suture(s) that are closed (Figure 11–2).

Craniosynostosis is a relatively common anomaly, occurring in about 1 in 1900 children. It comes to medical attention because the parents or the child's physician notices the abnormal skull shape. However, this is not the only reason for an infant to have an abnormal skull shape. In the immediate newborn period, it is common for infants born by vaginal delivery to have a tall, pointed skull. This is a result of the head molding to pass through the birth canal; and typically it will resolve over the course of a few days. It is not as common in infants born by Cesarean section.

Perhaps the most common reason for a child to have an abnormal skull shape is termed posterior positional plagiocephaly. Although the abnormal skull shape can be confused with that seen with true craniosynostosis, posterior positional plagiocephaly is not due to a premature fusion of a cranial suture. Rather, it is a result of an abnormal force that deforms the skull shape over the first few months of life (see Posterior Positional Plagiocephaly). Because the sutures remain patent, nonsurgical treatment is possible, whereas correction of true craniosynostosis requires surgical intervention.

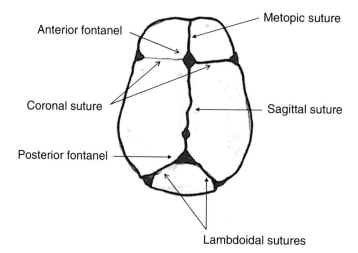

FIGURE 11–1. The normal shape of an infant skull, with patent sutures and fontanels

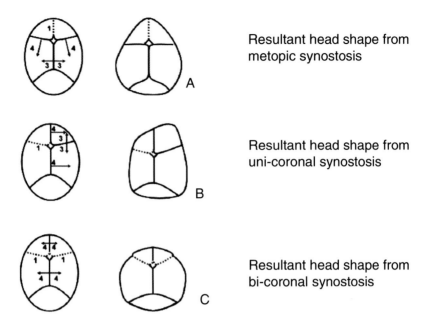

Resultant head shape from metopic synostosis

Resultant head shape from uni-coronal synostosis

Resultant head shape from bi-coronal synostosis

FIGURE 11–2. A–C. The abnormal head shapes seen due to premature closure of cranial suture(s) (see Figure 11–3 and Posterior Positional Plagiocephaly). (Adapted with permission from Orthomerica from *Post-Operative Treatment of Craniosynostosis* [White paper], by N. J. Igel, P. Stevens, D. Fish, and Lima, D, Sept. 2004.)

Posterior Positional Plagiocephaly

Posterior positional plagiocephaly is now among the most common indications for referral to craniofacial centers. The increase was noted soon after the "Back to Sleep" initiative put forth by the American Academy of Pediatrics in 1992. This recommendation was made in an effort to reduce the rate of sudden infant death syndrome (SIDS), and stated that all infants should be placed on their backs to sleep. Although this had the desired effect—there was a 40% reduction in the incidence of SIDS in the first few years of the program, from 1.17 per 1000 in 1993 to 0.53 per 1000 in 1987, it also had the unintended consequence of causing a sharp rise in the incidence of posterior positional plagiocephaly (Figure 11–3). Positional deformation results in an asymmetric head shape, with the occiput on one side becoming flatter than the other, pushing the ear on that side forward (toward the face), and the forehead on that

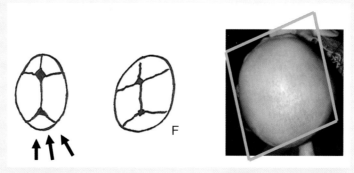

FIGURE 11–3. A young child with posterior positional plagiocephaly. This can be differentiated from true craniosynostosis by several findings: (1) the ear on the affected side is
displaced forward (toward the face); (2) there is compensa-
tory bulging of the forehead on the opposite side of the posterior bulging, resulting in a parallelogram head shape; and
(3) when severe and/or long-standing, facial asymmetry
may be seen as well. (Adapted with permission from
Orthomerica from *Post-Operative Treatment of Craniosynostosis* [White paper], by N. J. Igel, P. Stevens, D. Fish, and
Lima, D, Sept. 2004.)

side becoming more prominent. Once asymmetric, the infant's skull
will preferentially rest in that position, further deforming the skull.
The process stops once the infant gains head control and can move
his or her head independently. However, by that point, the skull may
be significantly asymmetric and, in severe and long-standing cases,
facial asymmetry can be seen as well.

The resultant skull shape with posterior positional plagiocephaly
can mimic that seen with unilateral lambdoidal craniosynostosis.
However, it is a different process and, therefore, has different
treatment options. Unlike true craniosynostosis, the sutures remain
patent in posterior positional plagiocephaly. For true craniosynostosis, surgical treatment is the only option to correct the abnormal
skull shape. With posterior positional plagiocephaly, the causative
process is of a limited duration. The subsequent normal growth that
occurs after head control is achieved will lessen the severity of the
asymmetry, so many cases do not require any treatment. This is
particularly true for those that are identified early, as active head
repositioning will limit progression. Although surgical intervention
rarely may be indicated for the most severe cases, molding helmets
have been used with much success. One such example is the
Orthomerica "Star Band" (Figure 11–4). Contraindications to this

treatment include the presence of true craniosynostosis, hydro-cephalus, and age below 3 months or over 18 months.

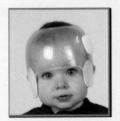 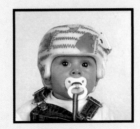

FIGURE 11–4. Nonsurgical treatments for posterior positional plagiocephaly include use of orthotic mold-ing helmets. For more information, please see http://www.Orthomeric.com.

PRIMARY VERSUS SECONDARY CRANIOSYNOSTOSIS

In evaluating a child with craniosynostosis, the initial step is to determine if the premature fusion is a primary or secondary event. Secondary craniosynostosis occurs as a consequence of diminished brain growth. In the normal state, the sutures remain patent early in life due to the pressure of the underlying growing brain. If the brain growth is not normal due to an acquired insult or genetic problem, the sutures will close prematurely. Secondary craniosynostosis results in a head that has a normal overall shape but small head circumference with possible ridging along the cranial sutures. Often these children manifest developmental delay and have other neurodevelopmental findings. An example of a genetic syndrome with secondary craniosynostosis is Seckel syndrome (Figure 11-5). This is an autosomal recessive disorder characterized by microcephaly, distinct beaked nose, marked short stature, and significant developmental delay.

Primary Craniosynostosis

Primary craniosynostosis implies that the early closure is due to an intrinsic abnormality of the skull bones or cranial sutures. This can be caused by either a primary genetic abnormality, such as a mutation in a gene encoding for a

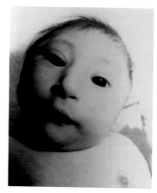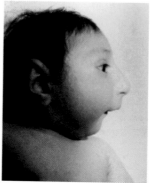

FIGURE 11–5. An infant with Seckel syndrome and craniosynostosis. Note the symmetric normal skull contour and microcephaly, indicating secondary craniosynostosis. (Reprinted with permission of Wiley-Liss, Inc. a subsidiary of John Wiley & Sons, Inc. from "Central Nervous System Anomalies in Seckel Syndrome: Report of a New Family and Review of the Literature," by A. Shanske, D. G. Caride, Menasse-Palmer, L., Bogdanow, A., and Marion, R. W., 1997. *American Journal of Medical Genetics, 70*(2),155–158.)

protein involved in cranial suture development, or an abnormality that is not primarily genetic. Examples include hyperthyroidism, torticollis (contracture of a neck muscle), and metabolic storage diseases, such as Hurler syndrome. In each, the underlying disease can cause the cranial sutures to fuse prematurely.

Craniosynostosis and Head Shape

Isolated Craniosynostosis

Like all other congenital anomalies, craniosynostosis can occur as part of a genetic syndrome, but it is much more commonly an isolated finding, in a child with no other anomalies. Isolated craniosynostosis is rarely familial, with the exact proportion of familial cases depending on which suture is involved.

There are four cranial sutures along the round portion of the calvarium (skull) (see Figure 11-1). The metopic and sagittal sutures are single, and course along the cranial midline. The coronal and lambdoidal sutures are in pairs. Premature closure of any of these sutures results in a distinctive skull shape (see Figure 11-2). The abnormal shape is symmetric if the metopic or sagittal sutures are involved, or if both coronal or lambdoidal sutures are closed. However, marked skull asymmetry is seen when one of the paired sutures is involved.

Sagittal craniosynostosis produces a scaphocephalic head shape (Figure 11–6), one that is elongated long anterior to posterior. It is the most common form of true craniosynostosis, accounting for 40 to 55% of all cases. Males are more than three times more commonly affected than females. Only about 5% of cases are familial, and in such cases sagittal craniosynostosis typically demonstrates an autosomal dominant pattern, with reduced penetrance—less than 40% of people who are obligate carriers of the trait will manifest sagittal craniosynostosis. The majority of cases are isolated, but about 25% of cases have associated anomalies.

Coronal craniosynostosis produces a head shape that is brachycephalic, a skull that is wide and short in the anterior to posterior dimension (Figure 11-7). The forehead typically is broad. Coronal craniosynostosis accounts for about 20 to 30% of all cases of apparently isolated craniosynostosis, but is the most common form of craniosynostosis that occurs in genetic syndromes. Interestingly, some of the gene mutations that cause the syndromic forms of coronal craniosynostosis can also cause isolated coronal craniosynostosis. About 35% of unilateral coronal craniosynostosis, and 47% of bilateral, is associated with other anomalies. Isolated coronal craniosynostosis is twice as common in females. Like sagittal, only a small fraction of isolated coronal craniosynostosis is familial, about 5 to 15%, and typically is inherited in an autosomal dominant pattern. Interestingly, there has been some association between the occurrence of coronal craniosynostosis and older paternal age (over 40 years old).

Premature fusion of the *metopic* suture causes the front of the skull to be narrowed and the back to be widened, giving the skull a triangular appearance when viewed from above (Figure 11-8). This is referred to as "trigonencephaly." Metopic craniosynostosis is relatively uncommon, accounting for 3 to 10% of all craniosynostosis. It is rarely familial, and is associated with other anomalies in fewer than 20% or cases. However, metopic craniosynostosis is a prominent manifestation in several genetic disorders, including Opitz C syndrome, and in deletions of chromosome 9p. Both are associated with significant neurodevelopmental delays and often other congenital anomalies.

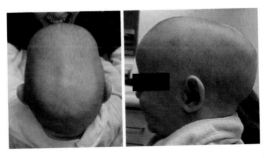

FIGURE 11–6. An infant with sagittal craniosynostosis. Note the elongated but symmetric skull shape. (Courtesy of John H Grant, M.D.)

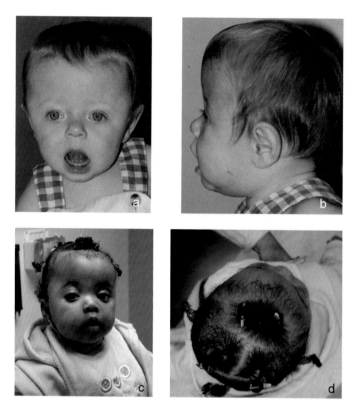

FIGURE 11–7. Bilateral coronal craniosynostosis. **A.** Note the wider skull shape in the frontal image and **B.** the narrow front to back distance. **C.** and **D.** Unicoronal craniosynostosis. Note the wide and asymmetric forehead (C), and the right forehead recessed (D). (Courtesy of John H. Grant, M.D.)

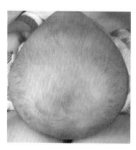

FIGURE 11–8. Metopic craniosynostosis. Note the triangular skull shape. (Courtesy of Orthomerica.)

Lambdoidal craniosynostosis is usually unilateral, resulting in an asymmetric skull shape ("plagiocephaly"). One sees flattening in the region of the closed suture, with bulging out on the opposite side of the occiput and ipsilateral frontal area. It is very common, but almost always occurs secondary to mechanical deformation, such as abnormal in-utero positioning, or torticollis.

SYNDROMIC CRANIOSYNOSTOSIS

Craniosynostosis occurs as one finding in over 150 genetic syndromes. In most instances, the associated anomalies are obvious, but in some cases they are subtle. Furthermore, an exact diagnosis often can be made only through identifying these minor anomalies. This is obviously necessary for parents to receive accurate counseling regarding not only recurrence risk but prognosis and etiology as well.

Most of the craniosynostosis syndromes are inherited as autosomal dominant traits, with variable expression. Although it is impossible to review, or even list, all of these syndromes, we will review a select number, including the well-known craniosynostosis syndromes, such as Apert and Crouzon syndromes, but also less well-known disorders, such as craniofrontonasal syndrome and Muenke syndrome (Figure 11-9). The molecular genetic basis for many of these syndromes has been recently uncovered. Although these discoveries have provided new insights into these syndromes as well as normal and abnormal craniofacial development, they have also revealed fascinating if sometimes unexpected results.

Apert, Crouzon, and Related Syndromes

Apert syndrome is one of the classic craniosynostosis syndromes (Table 11-1), a group that includes Crouzon, Pfeiffer, Saethre-Chotzen, Jackson-Weiss, and the relatively newly identified Muenke syndromes. These are among the earliest recognized known genetic syndromes, with some dating back to the mid-19th century. These syndromes share many characteristics, both clinical and genetic. Although many cases occur with no family history, all are autosomal dominant disorders, with complete penetrance and variable expressivity.

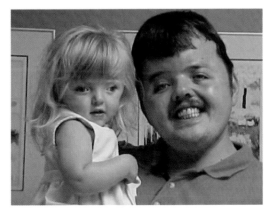

FIGURE 11–9. Father and daughter with Muenke syndrome (FGFR3-related coronal craniosynostosis).

TABLE 11–1. The Clinical Characteristics of the Common Craniosynostosis Syndromes. All manifest the common craniofacial findings of coronal craniosynostosis, midface hypoplasia with ocular proptosis, beaked nose, small mouth with high arched palate, and dental crowding.

Syndrome	Limb Findings	Additional Findings	Gene(s) (Mutation)
Crouzon syndrome	None[a]	None	FGFR2 (many)
Crouzon syndrome with acanthosis nigricans	None[a]	Acanthosis nigricans	FGFR3
Pfeiffer syndrome			
Type I	Broad and medially deviated thumbs and great toes; short fingers and toes	None	FGFR1 (Pro252Arg); FGFR2 (many)
Type II	Same as Type I, plus ankylosis (fusion) of the elbows, other joints	Cloverleaf skull; upper airway anomalies (choanal stenosis, tracheal rings); severe neurologic impairment; early death is common	FGFR2 (many)
Type III	Same as Type II	Same as Type II, except the cloverleaf skull is not present	FGFR2 (many)
Jackson-Weiss syndrome	Broad and medially deviated great toes, normal hands	None	FGFR2 (many)
Apert syndrome	Mitten glove syndactyly of fingers and toes	Cleft palate (occasional)	FGFR2 (many)
Beare-Stevenson with cutis gyrata	Ankylosis (fusion) of the elbows	Cutis gyrate (excessive skin folds); prominent umbilical stump; anterior anus; hydrocephalus, developmental delay	FGFR2 (many)

TABLE 11–1. *continued*

Syndrome	Limb Findings	Additional Findings	Gene(s) (Mutation)
Saethre-Chotzen	Broad and laterally deviated great toes, normal hands	Ptosis; developmental delay (especially with large deletions)	TWIST (point mutations and deletions)
Muenke syndrome	Variable—normal, broad thumbs and great toes, short fingers and toes[b]	Variable—hearing impairment, isolated macrocephaly	FGFR3 (Pro250Arg)
Nonsyndromic craniosynostosis (NSC)	None	None	FGFR2 (many); FGFR3 (Pro250Arg)

[a]By x-ray the bones of the hands and feet may be small.
[b]Carpal-tarsal fusion may be seen on x-ray.

These syndromes also share a similar craniofacial appearance. This includes turribrachcephaly due to coronal craniosynostosis; widely spaced eyes that are often proptotic due to underdevelopment of the bony orbits; a small beaked nose; and small mouth with a high palate and dental crowding. Although each has a slightly different rate of complications such as mental retardation, cleft palate, and hearing loss, these syndromes classically have been distinguished by their particular hand and foot findings (Figure 11-10). However, recent research has shown that these subtle clinical differences are not reflected by the underlying genetic basis for these syndromes.

Fibroblast Growth Factor Receptor and TWIST Mutations in Syndromic and Nonsyndromic Craniosynostosis

Crouzon, Pfeiffer, Apert, Jackson-Weiss, and Muenke syndromes are each caused by mutations in a *fibroblast growth factor receptor (FGFR)* gene. *FGFRs* are a family of four (*FGFR1-4*) genes that code for cell surface receptors that bind fibroblast growth factors (*FGF*), and function to regulate cell proliferation, differentiation, and migration through a variety of complex pathways. A single mutation in *FGFR1* (Figure 11-11A) (substitution of a proline for arginine at amino acid position 250; Pro250Arg) causes Pfeiffer syndrome, although a variety of different mutations in *FGFR2* (Figure 11-11B) can cause either Pfeiffer, Apert, Crouzon, or Jackson-Weiss syndromes, and mutations in *FGFR3* (Figure 11-11C) cause Muenke syndrome, and a form of Crouzon syndrome associated with a skin disorder, acanthosis nigricans. Mutations in both

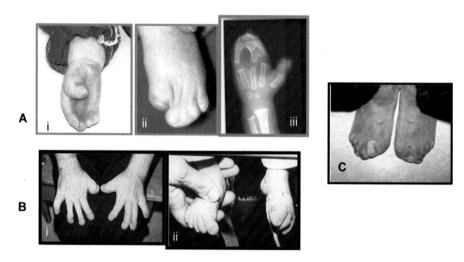

FIGURE 11–10. The hand and foot findings of the craniosynostosis syndromes **A.** Mitten glove syndactyly of Apert syndrome. Note the bone syndactyly in A-iii. **B.** Broad and medially deviated thumbs and great toes of Pfeiffer syndrome. **C.** Broad and laterally deviated thumbs and great toes of Saethre-Chotzen syndrome.

FGFR2 and *FGFR3* have been associated with nonsyndromic craniosynostosis as well, and the *FGFR3* mutation that causes Muenke syndrome (also Pro250Arg) has also been associated with other clinical presentations, including nonsyndromic hearing impairment (DFNA13, see Chapter 9), isolated macrocephaly, and even normal. Other mutations in *FGFR3* cause achondroplasia, a common cause of dwarfism, and several other skeletal disorders (Figure 11–12; see Achondroplasia). *FGFR1-3* are expressed in developing skeletal tissue, and their normal function is to restrain limb growth. The mutations associated with these syndromes are "hypermorphic," they make the protein work too well. Saethre Chotzen syndrome is caused by mutations in a different gene, TWIST. In contrast to the FGFR mutations, the TWIST mutation that causes Saethre Chotzen knocks out the protein's function.

Genetic testing for all of the craniosynostosis syndromes is available on a clinical basis through a number of laboratories. However, the chance of detecting a mutation is far from certain. Depending on the clinical diagnosis, the rate of positive tests ranges from about 50% for Crouzon syndrome to over 90% for clinically classic Apert syndrome. (Note: the detection rate for Muenke syndrome is more than 99%, as it is defined by the presence of the Pro250Arg mutation in FGFR3.) The primary benefits of genetic testing for syndromic craniosynostosis are to identify a marker that will facilitate prenatal testing for future offspring, and to confirm the diagnosis. Prognosis and management decisions can be effectively gauged by a clinical diagnosis, as there is limited additional information that correlates to a specific genotype. However, this is not the case for isolated craniosynostosis, or patients who

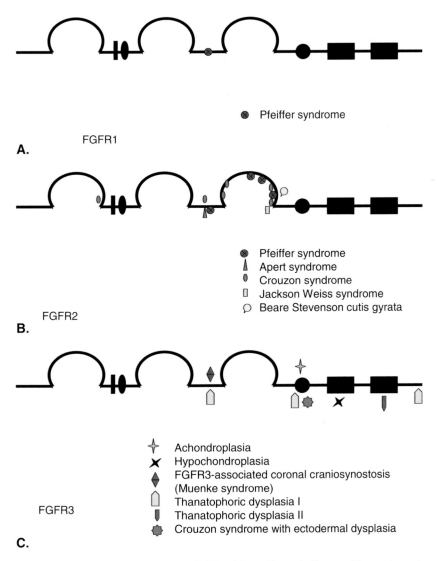

A. FGFR1

● Pfeiffer syndrome

B. FGFR2

⊗ Pfeiffer syndrome
▲ Apert syndrome
◗ Crouzon syndrome
▯ Jackson Weiss syndrome
◯ Beare Stevenson cutis gyrata

C. FGFR3

✦ Achondroplasia
✗ Hypochondroplasia
◆ FGFR3-associated coronal craniosynostosis
   (Muenke syndrome)
▯ Thanatophoric dysplasia I
▯ Thanatophoric dysplasia II
❂ Crouzon syndrome with ectodermal dysplasia

FIGURE 11–11. A depiction of Fibroblast Growth Factor Receptors 1 (**A**), 2 (**B**), and 3 (**C**), showing the general location of the known disease-related mutations for the craniosynostosis syndromes: Pfeiffer, Apert, Crouzon, Jackson-Weiss, FGFR3-associated coronal craniosynostosis (Muenke), and Beare-Stevenson cutis gyrata. Also shown are the mutations associated with several skeletal dysplasia: Achondroplasia, Hypochondroplasia, and Thanatophoric dysplasia types 1 and 2. A more detailed discussion of these conditions can be found at http://www.geneclinics.org

have no other anomalies. This is an important distinction to make, as many patients with coronal with or without other suture synostosis will have other anomalies that, although they do not comprise one of the classic recognized

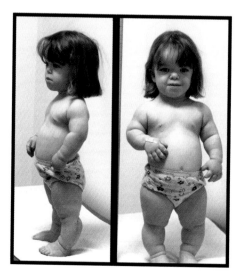

FIGURE 11–12. A 3-year-old girl with achondroplasia. Note the relatively large skull, midface underdevelopment, and limbs that are short, but most affected in the proximal segment (so-called "rhizomelia").

syndrome, are still likely to have an FGFR or TWIST mutation as the underlying cause of their phenotype.

For truly isolated craniosynostosis, however, genetic testing is much less likely to identify a causative mutation. For sagittal, metopic, and lambdoidal synostosis the likelihood is so low that testing is not recommended, but this is not the case for isolated coronal synostosis. Although the detection rates are low, mutations in FGFR2, FGFR3, or TWIST have been identified in patients with isolated uni- or bicoronal craniosynostosis. These results have significance for several reasons. First, identifying a mutation permits a more accurate recurrence risk to be defined. If a parent carries the same mutation, the risk is 50%, whereas it is less than 1% if neither parents carries the mutation. Mutation testing also can provide at least limited prognostic information as well. The risk for other medical problems, such as dental anomalies and hearing loss, is higher in mutation-positive patients. Furthermore, patients with an FGFR3 mutation have been shown in small studies to have a five- to seven-fold higher rate of requiring a second cranial operation to correct a functional impairment, compared to 4% in patients without an FGFR3 mutation. For this reason, many advocate genetic testing for all patients with coronal craniosynostosis, even those with no suggesting family history or other physical findings. It is of paramount importance that such testing be done in conjunction with genetic evaluation and counseling, so that an exact diagnosis can be reached, and families can fully understand the benefits and limitations of this testing. For a more detailed discussion of the testing issues, the reader is referred to entries on FGFR-related syndromes at http://www.Genereviews.org.

Achondroplasia

Achondroplasia is the most common genetic form of short stature. It is a generalized skeletal dysplasia that results in disproportionately short arms and legs, a relatively large head, and characteristic facial features that resemble these seen in the FGFR-related cranio-synostosis syndromes. This includes frontal bossing, wide-set eyes, mid-face hypoplasia, and a small mouth. Conductive hearing loss is very common due to an abnormal skull base and associated Eustachian tube dysfunction. In addition, upper airway obstruction and/or sleep apnea can occur, either due to anatomic problems or secondary to spinal cord compression due to a narrow foramen magnum (the opening at the base of the skull through which the spinal cord passes). This requires immediate medical and often surgical management.

Achondroplasia is inherited as an autosomal dominant trait. About 80% of cases are the result of a new mutation, with both parents having normal stature. In the remaining 20% of cases one parent has achondroplasia. A person with achondroplasia is at 50% chance for having a child with achondroplasia, 50% chance for having a child of normal stature. If both parents have achondroplasia (a relatively common occurrence), there is still a 50% chance that they will have a child with achondroplasia, but only a 25% chance for a child of normal stature. The last possible outcome is that both parents will pass down their mutant FGFR3 gene so that the fetus has two copies. This risk is also 25%, and results in a lethal condition called homozygous achondroplasia.

Achondroplasia is caused by a specific mutation in the gene fibroblast growth factor receptor (FGFR) 3. The normal FGFR3 protein acts to slow down bone growth during development, and this mutation causes the protein to work too well. Clinical testing is available, but the diagnosis can usually be made based on clinical findings.

Other Craniofacial Syndromes

Below is a brief review of several syndromes that are relatively common or well known, or are mistaken for syndromes that are more common or well known. This is of course a *very* limited list—several hundred genetics syndromes have craniofacial findings. For more a more extensive list, with more detailed information, the reader is referred to any one of several excellent texts that are listed at the end of the chapter.

Baller Gerold Syndrome

This syndrome is characterized by craniosynostosis and radial aplasia. Cranio-synostosis usually involves the coronal sutures but may involve other sutures as well. The radial defect is typically bilateral, but it may be asymmetric, resulting in radial absence on one side and a milder underdevelopment on the other (Figure 11–13). The thumb may be absent, and the ulna is typically short and curved. There may be associated craniofacial findings, such as hypertelorism, epicanthic folds, a prominent nasal bridge, midline capillary hemangiomas, genitourinary malformations, and developmental delay/mental retardation. Inheritance has been thought to be autosomal recessive, but heterozygous (e.g., autosomal dominant) mutations in the TWIST gene have been identified in some individuals with Baller-Gerold syndrome. As mutations in TWIST are associated with Saethre-Chotzen syndrome, this raises the possibility that, at least in some cases, the Baller-Gerold phenotype is another manifestation of Saethre-Chotzen syndrome.

Wildervank Syndrome

This is a rare autosomal dominant condition that can be mistaken for oculoauriculovertebral spectrum, as it can present with hemifacial microsomia and preauricular skin tags and pits. It is differentiated from oculoauriculovertebral spectrum by the presence of multiple fused cervical vertebrae resulting in a short neck with limited movement (so called "Klippel-Feil" anomaly), sensorineural hearing impairment, and Duane syndrome (absence of cranial nerve VI, preventing the eye from lateral gaze). Duane syndrome can also be seen in oculoauriculovertebral spectrum (see Chapter 5).

Romberg (or Parry Romberg) Syndrome

This is another disorder that can be mistaken for oculoauriculovertebral spectrum. However, it is much less common, and has a very different natural history. Affected individuals are born with a normal face, but sometime in the first decade of life experience a progressive atrophy (wasting away) of the soft tissue on one side of the face (Figure 11–14). The tongue, soft palate, and gums may also be affected, and skeletal growth is typically retarded as well, giving

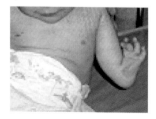

FIGURE 11–13. Radial ray hypoplasia, as seen in Baller Gerold syndrome.

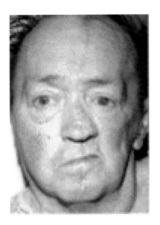

FIGURE 11–14. Parry Romberg syndrome. Note that the entire left side of the face is smaller and more darkly pigmented. The right side is spared. Also note the demarcation of the midline. (Reprinted courtesy of Postgraduate Medicine from "Rare Cause of Facial Asymmetry. Progressive Facial Hemiatrophy," by Y. Y. Mishriki, 2005. *Postgraduate Medicine, 117*(4), 40, 43–44.)

the appearance of hemifacial microsomia. The cause of Romberg syndrome is not known, but there is no evidence of an underlying genetic basis.

Frontonasal Dysplasia

Frontal dysplasia is another common anomaly that is etiologically heterogeneous. It is characterized by hypertelorism and a broad nasal tip that has either a central dimple or longitudinal groove. A "widow's peak" (a "V"-shaped point formed by hair at the center of the anterior hairline) may be seen as well. Frontonasal dysplasia has a variety of causes, including chromosomal imbalances, single gene syndromes, maternal diabetes, or a nasal encephalocele. Most cases are isolated, associated with normal intelligence and no other birth defects. In any case, the underlying problem is one where the nasal placode is not formed, permitting the developing forebrain to protrude forward and hinder the medial migration of the lateral facial structures, including the eyes.

One syndrome that manifests frontonasal dysplasia, which is very rare but very interesting, is **craniofrontonasal syndrome**. This is a unique X-linked disorder, unique because females are *more* severely affected than males. Associated findings that are more common in females include coronal craniosynostosis, facial asymmetry, cleft palate, and a mild ectodermal dysplasia manifesting as ridging of the fingernails and brittle hair. Males typically have mild facial findings. The gene for craniofronotonasal syndrome is EFNB1, on the X chromosome. Although much research has focused on explaining this exceptional inheritance pattern, it is still not yet known.

Greig Cephalopolysyndactyly Syndrome

This is a very variable autosomal dominant disorder characterized by the finding of extra fingers and/or toes, hypertelorism, and macrocephaly with a broad and prominent forehead. The cranial appearance can be mistaken for coronal craniosynostosis, which is not common in Greig cephalopolysyndactyly syndrome. The extra digits can be either on the "thumb" side ("preaxial" polydactyly), "pinky" side ("postaxial" polydactyly), or "mixed," with both pre- and postaxial polydactyly. Greig cephalopolysyndactyly syndrome is caused by alteration in the gene GLI3. About 30% are deletions, which are detected by cytogenetics, FISH, or CGH; the rest are mutations identified through gene sequencing. Patients with deletions are more likely to manifest developmental delay and seizures. Different mutations in GLI3 can cause the more mild phenotype of isolated form of polydactyly (polydactyly type A4), or the more severe Pallister Hall syndrome.

Treacher Collins Syndrome

Treacher Collins syndrome is an autosomal dominant disorder characterized by hypoplasia of the maxilla, especially the zygoma, creating a distinct facial appearance (Figure 11–15). Other key clinical findings include down-slanting palpebral fissures, absence of the lower eyelashes, lower eyelid coloboma, small auricles, and micrognathia. More severely affected individuals may require a tracheostomy due to the small airway. It is an autosomal dominant disorder, with about 60% of cases being the result of a new mutation. However, the physical findings may be very mild, so an affected parent may not be unrecognized. Treacher Collins syndrome is caused by mutations in the gene TREACLE, on chromosome 5q32.

Nager syndrome has a similar facial appearance as Treacher Collins, but is differentiated by the presence of preaxial (radial) limb anomalies, including hypoplasia or absence of the thumbs and radii. Most cases are new mutations, but, like Treacher Collins, it can be inherited as an autosomal dominant trait. The specific gene has not yet been identified.

Opitz G Syndrome

Also called Opitz BBB, and Opitz Frias J syndrome, Opitz G syndrome has a distinct facial appearance—a widow's peak, wide set eyes ("hypertelorism"), broad upturned nose, and cleft lip with or without a cleft palate (Figure 11–16). Other defects include hypospadias (the urethra opens on the ventral [underside] surface of the penis), posterior pharyngeal cleft (which can lead to aspiration), imperforate anus, and congenital heart defects. Mental retardation/developmental delay can be seen, as can anatomic brain anomalies. Opitz G syndrome is genetically heterogeneous, with X-linked and autosomal dominant forms. The X-linked type is more common. It is caused by mutations in the gene MID1. Females are mildly affected, and may only manifest hypertelorism or the widow's peak, whereas males typically have a more classic phenotype. The autosomal dominant form of Opitz G maps is uncommon, with only sev-

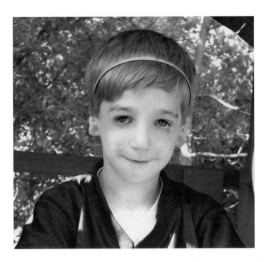

FIGURE 11–15. A young boy with Treacher Collins syndrome. Note the maxillary hypoplasia, lower eyelid defects, and malformed ears.(Courtesy of the Treacher Collins support group, "Treacher Collins Connect" [http://www.tcconnection.org].)

eral families being reported. Phenotypically, it is essentially identical to that of the X-linked form, but the present of male-to-male transmission of the condition in these families eliminates the possibility of X-linked inheritance and supports an autosomal dominant inheritance. The gene maps to a segment of chromosome 22q, overlapping the locus for del22q11 (velocardiofacial syndrome). Reports have suggested that the autosomal dominant form of Opitz G was another variant of del22q11/velocardiofacial syndrome. However, the cases of Opitz G that mapped to chromosome 22q did not have the 22q11 deletion. It is more likely that autosomal dominant Opitz G is a separate entity from del22q11/velocardiofacial syndrome, and that some cases of del22q11 can have findings that suggest Opitz G syndrome, such as hypertelorism and hypospadias. This is an important distinction, as individuals who have a clinical appearance of Opitz G but test positive for the 22q11 deletion must be managed as if they have del22q11/ velocardiofacial syndrome, not as if they have Opitz G.

Several other syndromes have hypertelorism as a prominent finding. Each has a facial appearance that is distinctive to a trained geneticist, but would be hard to differentiate in the absence of experience with these syndromes. These syndromes include: **Aarskog syndrome**, an X-linked disorder in which affected males have short stature, small hands, and a shawl scrotum (the gene is called FGD1) and **Robinow syndrome**, which has both autosomal dominant and autosomal recessive forms (Figure 11–17A). It is characterized by short stature, short limbs, and a small phallus in males. The autosomal

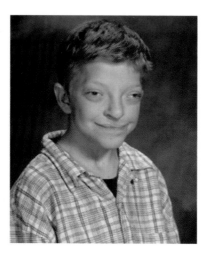

FIGURE 11–16. A young man with Opitz G syndrome. Note the wide-set eyes and broad nose.

recessive form is caused by mutations in the gene ROR2. Individuals who are heterozygote for this mutation (e.g., parents of affected children), have Brachydactyly B, a form of short fingers. The autosomal recessive form of Robinow syndrome is more severe than the autosomal dominant form, as it typically associated with other birth defects and significant developmental delay; **Coffin Lowry syndrome** is an X-linked disorder that is characterized by short stature and severe developmental delay in affected males (Figure 11–17B). The underlying cause is mutations in the gene RSK2. The facial appearance of Coffin Lowry syndrome is characterized by sallow cheeks and a wide mouth with full lips. This is similar to that seen in **Williams syndrome**. However, they are very different disorders (see p. 46 in Chapter 4).

Sotos Syndrome

This syndrome is characterized by overgrowth (macrocephaly and increased height), a distinct facial appearance (long face, prominent chin, hypertelorism), and variable developmental delay (Figure 11–18). There are often associated problems, such as seizures, strabismus, conductive hearing loss, congenital heart defects, renal anomalies, and behavioral problems. with neonatal jaundice, scoliosis, seizures, There is also a slightly increased risk for certain tumors, such as sacrococcygeal teratoma and neuroblastoma. Radiographic studies will reveal an advanced bone age, and head imaging will show enlarged ventricles. This is not, however, due to hydrocephalus. Sotos syndrome is caused by alterations in the gene NDS1. In the United States and Europe, about 10% of

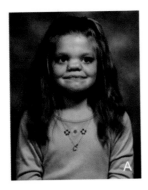
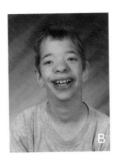

FIGURE 11–17. **A.** Picture of a girl with Robinow syndrome Courtesy of the Robinow Syndrome Foundation. **B.** Picture of a boy with Coffin-Lowry syndrome. (Reprinted with permission of Wiley-Liss, Inc. a subsidiary of John Wiley & Sons, Inc. from "Cardiomyopathy in Coffin-Lowry Syndrome," by Facher et al., 2004. *American Journal of Medical Genetics, 28*(2), 176–178.)

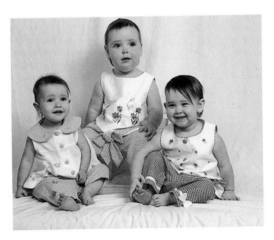

FIGURE 11–18. A young girl with Sotos syndrome (*middle*). She is flanked by her triplet sisters. Note her larger size and longer face.

cases will have a microdeletion of this gene detectable by FISH studies, while more than 75% will have a point mutation that requires sequence analysis. Interestingly, in Japan, where NDS1 alterations were first identified in Sotos syndrome, FISH deletions are found in about 50% of cases.

RECOMMENDED READING

Doherty, E. S., & Muenke, M. (2006). *Muenke syndrome.* GeneClinics: Medical Genetics Knowledge Base [database online]. Copyright, University of Washington, Seattle. Updated weekly. Available at http://www.geneclinics.org.

Gorlin, R. J., Cohen, M,. Jr., & Hennekam, R. C. M. (Eds.). (2001). *Syndromes of the head and neck* (4th ed.). Oxford Monographs on Medical Genetics. New York: Oxford University Press.

Mulliken, J. B., Gripp, K. W., Stolle, C. A., Steinberger, D., & Muller, U. (2004). Molecular analysis of patients with synostotic frontal plagiocephaly (unilateral coronal synostosis). *Plastic and Reconstructive Surgery, 113*(7), 1899–1909.

Robin, N. H., & Falk, M. J. (2006). *FGFR-related craniosynostosis.* GeneClinics: Medical Genetics Knowledge Base [database online]. Copyright, University of Washington, Seattle. 1995–. Updated weekly. Available at http://www.geneclinics.org.

Stevenson, R. E., & Hall, J. G. (2006) *Human malformations and related anomalies* (2nd ed., Pt. IV, chaps. 7 & 8). New York: Oxford University Press.

Thomas, G. P., Wilkie, A. O., Richards, P. G., & Wall, S. A.. (2005). FGFR3 P250R mutation increases the risk of reoperation in apparent "nonsyndromic" coronal craniosynostosis. *Journal of Craniofacial Surgery, 16*(3), 347–352.

Index